An Introduction
to the
Ethos of Nursing

An Introduction to the Ethos of Nursing

A text for basic student nurses

JOYCE MARY MELLISH
DN(Wits), BA(SA), MCur(Ed), MCur(Admin), D Cur(Pret), RNA, RM, RCN, RT,
Emeritus Professor of Nursing Science
University of Port Elizabeth

Butterworths
Durban

© 1988
Butterworth Publishers (Pty) Ltd
Reg No 70/02642/07

ISBN 0 409 10007 2

THE BUTTERWORTH GROUP

South Africa
BUTTERWORTH PUBLISHERS (PTY) LTD
8 Walter Place, Waterval Park, Mayville, Durban 4091

England
BUTTERWORTH & CO (PUBLISHERS) LTD
London

Australia
BUTTERWORTHS (PTY) LTD
Sydney   Melbourne   Brisbane   Adelaide   Perth

Canada
BUTTERWORTHS CANADA
Toronto Vancouver

New Zealand
BUTTERWORTHS OF NEW ZEALAND LTD
Wellington Auckland

Singapore
BUTTERWORTH & CO (ASIA) PTE LTD
Singapore

United States of America
BUTTERWORTH LEGAL PUBLISHERS
Austin   Boston   St Paul   Seattle
D & S PUBLISHERS INC
Clearwater Florida

Typeset by Positone, Pinetown.
Printed by Interpak Natal, Pietermarizburg

Preface

Nursing in the Republic of South Africa has undergone further extensive changes since the appearance of *Ethos of Nursing 2nd edition* in 1985, and these have necessitated a total revamping of the work.

The result is *An Introduction to the Ethos of Nursing, A text for basic student nurses*. In this book material that is now readily available in other sources has been drastically pruned to make way for important new material such as new ideas and changes in nursing education, and the functioning of the SANC and SANA.

I am extremely grateful to Una Brown, an ex-student of mine, who gave up many hours of her time to assist with the preparation of this text.

Acknowledgement must also go to Professor CK Oberholzer for guidance during the lectures and discussion sessions which are part of the study for the MCur degree. This contributed much to the clarification of my thoughts on nursing and what it is.

Finally, I acknowledge with gratitude the assistance and guidance of Professor C Searle during the years that I was one of her students.

JOYCE MARY MELLISH
Cape Town
1988

Challenges

During the study of this book it is suggested that the following are considered:
1 List and discuss the specific ethical dilemmas that may be faced by nurses dealing with persons in the following age groups:
   - neonates (1-6 weeks)
   - infants (6 weeks to 1 year)
   - children (1–11 years)
   - adolescents (11–18 years)
   - young adults (18–25 years)
   - adults (25–35 years)
   - middlescents (35–65 years)
   - the elderly (>65 years)

   This classification varies according to demographic variables. In each instance state the ethical principle involved, for example rights, veracity, etc.
2 You have been asked to address a group of second year student nurses on the subject 'Science deals with what is . . . Ethics deals with what ought to be'. Give an outline of your talk.
3 A neonate, born to a couple who are Jehovah's Witnesses, urgently needs an exchange of blood because of Rh incompatibility. The doctor advises treatment but the parents refuse to agree to it. What course of action do you think the doctor will take? Why? What ethical principle is involved? What is the duty of the nurse under such circumstances?
4 Analyse the South African Nurses' Pledge of Service. Think about and discuss the meaning and implications for nursing practice of each of the words of the pledge of service.
5 You are a member of a specific cultural group which has its own norms regarding health practices and care. Enumerate these. Consider two other cultural groups with whom you come into contact. Determine the health norms of each of these cultures and compare them with your own and with each other. What implications does such an exercise have for nursing practice?
6 The diabetic foot of a Muslim patient is amputated in the operating theatre. The relatives arrive to claim the limb. Why would they do so, and what are the implications for nursing practice?

Contents

	Page
Preface	v
Challenges	vii

1 Ethos of nursing: the character or nature of nursing — 1

Ethos – what is it?	1
The study of the ethos of nursing	1
Nursing – what is it?	2
Man – the recipient of nursing	5
Disruption caused by illness	5
The one who nurses	5
Acceptance of the patient	6
Indispensable role of the nurse	6
The trust relationship	7
The world of the sick person	7
The threat of illness	7
Danger of depersonalisation	8
Availability of the nurse	8
Various definitions	9
Symbolism of the lamp	10
Theories of nursing	11

2 Evolution of nursing: historical trends — 12

Ethos – the character and nature	12
The effect of various factors on the evolution of nursing	13
Contribution of various groups to the evolution of nursing in South Africa	25

3 Nature and evolution of specific types of nursing — 39

General nursing	39
Midwifery	40
Psychiatric nursing	49
Community nursing	52
Primary health care – the role of the nurse	60
Privatisation	66
Specialisation in nursing	66

4 The profession of nursing — 70

Professionalism	70
Composition of the nursing profession in South Africa	82
A professional association	84

		Page
5	**Principles of professional practice in nursing**	89
	Legal aspects	89
	The independent, interdependent and dependent functions of a nurse ..Autonomoia... Role.	91
	The South African Nursing Council (SANC)	93
	The South African Nursing Association	97
	Other points of importance in professional practice	101
6	**The ethical basis of the profession of nursing**	104
	The origin of ethics as a science	104
	Professional ethics	106
	Clarification of ethical concepts	108
	A philosophical approach	109
	Ethical problems in the practice of nursing	110
	Conflicts in the work situation	117
7	**The concept 'duty'**	131
	Duty to fellow men	131
	Attitude of mind	136
	Compassion	137
	Active promotion of a state of well-being	137
	Conflict of duty	138
8	**Accountability**	140
	To whom is the nurse accountable?	140
	For what is the nurse accountable?	142
	General comments	145
9	**Discipline in the nursing context**	148
	The discipline of nursing	148
10	**Some other aspects of nursing**	156
	Nursing administration	156
	Nursing education	160
11	**The concept 'health' in the nursing context**	171
	Sickness and society	172
	Medical crises and the nurse	174
	Chronic illness and the nurse	175
	The rights and responsibilities of the nurse	175

	Page
Appendices	177
A The Hippocratic Oath	177
B Practical implications of the Health Act for Nursing	177
C The National Health Plan	181
D Codes of nursing ethics	184
E Criteria for brain death	187
F Ethical guidelines	188
Bibliography	191
Index	193

1 Ethos of nursing: the character or nature of nursing

ETHOS – WHAT IS IT?

The term 'ethos' is often used without much understanding of what is implied by it. The word 'ethos' is derived from the Greek and means the character or nature of an object. Thus this book deals with the character or nature of nursing. This is a wide concept comprising the meaning of nursing, the composition of the profession, the factors that brought it into being and the forces that moulded it, as well as the special characteristics and the norms of the group. In other words, the ethos of nursng is concerned with the existence of a total subculture of society.

The ethos of nursing is also concerned with the evolution, the development and the expansion of nursing – with the past, the present and the future. It shows the professional nurse where she has been, points out where she is now, and indicates the road into the future. It links nurses, from the primitive mother who gave care when necessary to the best of her ability and within the limitations of her knowledge, to the modern professional nurse, who also gives care to the best of her ability and within the limitation of the knowledge of today. The space-age nurse is a far cry from the primitive mother, but through the ages a chain has been forged which stretches into the future.

Tomorrow's abilities may well be more than today's, and tomorrow's knowledge will supersede that of today. The thread woven through the chain is the need for a specific type of care, irrespective of race, colour or creed. This care is given by the nurse.

The ethos of nursing is not the history of nursing, but it includes the study of that history. It is not ethics, but it includes the study of ethical concepts applied to nursing. It is not the theory and practice of nursing, but it includes the study of all aspects relating to nursing theory and practice. It is all-embracing.

THE STUDY OF THE ETHOS OF NURSING

How, then, does one go about studying such a vast subject? How does one assess the character of the profession? It will be necessary to decide what nursing is and what a profession is, and to understand the concepts of the professional practice related to nursing.

The development of nursing must be studied. The why, when, where, how, who and what must be looked at. The role played by history must be examined, the emphasis on trends that have affected the evolution and development of nursing. The ethical foundations of nursing must receive attention, as must the ethical problems that confront nurses. This work will attempt to provide guidelines for the study of the ethos of nursing. No work can do justice to the whole subject in one volume. The aim of this book will be to give a broad introduction, to arouse interest and stimulate inquiry upon which an in-depth study can be built.

NURSING – WHAT IS IT?

Nursing must have existed for as long as man himself – from the birth of the first helpless baby, from the time that the first man became unwell or was injured.

Nursing is a human activity

Because it concerns man, nursing is a human activity that takes place between members of the human race. It embraces a specific body of knowledge concerning man through all the phases of his life, from before conception until death. However, nursing is not concerned only with the sick person, but also with the healthy person, in which case the nurse's concern is to keep him healthy and functioning optimally in society as a human being who has physical, mental and social needs.

Nursing is unique

Nursing is not directed only at cure, but also includes promotive, preventive, rehabilitative and maintenance aspects. It is, therefore, a comprehensive concept.

Nursing is unique unto itself and must strive to remain so without stagnating. However, it is closely related to medical and other health care practices, but differs from each of them.

Nursing is part of health care

Nursing forms an essential component of a team approach to health care and recognises the value of the contribution of *all* health care professionals in meeting the specific health care needs demonstrated or expressed by the human being who is a patient or client.

Nursing is interpersonal in nature

Nursing, as a human phenomenon, is a specific type of behaviour among human beings. It is interpersonal in nature, for it exists only through interaction between human beings. Someone needs the nurse's care and she or he is ready and prepared to give the necessary nursing care. Machines and computers do not nurse, they only assist the persons, the nurses, who do.

A nurse interacts with her patients or clients, with her nursing colleagues, and with those colleagues who form the health team. Nursing does not occur in isolation, nor in a sterile laboratory atmosphere; there must be at least one human being, a patient or client, who has a human need which is met by another human being, the nurse, in a human way. This is a specific type of human need which the nurse, also a human being, is able to meet because of her preparation or education for the role. The human being in need of nursing care needs not only that specific care, but also the specific human being who can provide the care. The person, a patient or client, literally or figuratively calls upon someone who can and will listen to his need, interpret and understand it, and react positively to it. The person in need calls upon someone with the specific knowledge and skill to recognise the need for what it is, someone who will meet the need by taking specific, appropriate action.

Nursing is practical

Nursing is essentially *practical* in nature. The nurse uses her unique skills and knowledge to deliberately intervene in a situation in order to bring about a change. She also uses this special knowledge and these skills to prevent illness from occurring.

Nursing requires scientific knowledge

Nursing also has a *theoretical* side, for the practical application of nursing care is based on theoretical knowledge gleaned from the natural and social sciences, on medicine (an applied science) and on nursing itself. Man applies this theoretical knowledge in a practical way through nursing actions.

Science does not exist in sealed packages, for the development of scientific knowledge is the work of a person or of teams of people. The advances made in the various scientific fields were and are the result of the work of men. Ideas that lead to future discoveries first occur in the minds of men. *Knowledge is more than information,* for it requires experience and understanding. Information is stored in books or in computer memories. Knowledge, on the other hand, requires the ability of a human being to apply information to specific work, to action or to performance. When information remains confined to books and other storage facilities and the mind is not applied to using it, it is of limited value. Only when it is retrieved by human beings, analysed and used as the basis for human actions, mental or physical, does information become knowledge.

Nursing is a human science

Above all nursing science is a *human science* which has its origins in a specific facet of the life world of man, a facet that is part of human existence, part of 'being human'. It originates in the very existence of man and is an inseparable part of it. The science of nursing has not developed from discoveries in a laboratory, although, like all sciences, it uses such discoveries.

Nursing is an art

Nursing is not only a science but also an art, and in the practice of her nursing science the nurse sees the individual together with the organic, physiological or psychological problems that have brought him into the sphere of nursing care.

Nursing is caring

The word 'caring', from the old English *caru*, means to be concerned about or interested in, to have regard for, to show solicitude for.

In the course of her work the nurse is concerned about or shows solicitude for the person in need of nursing. This can take the form of physical caring, of doing for the person (patient) what he is unable to do for himself, temporarily or permanently. In attending to physical needs the caring nurse will consider the feelings of the recipient of care and preserve his dignity. While a person may willingly strip in front of other people, the effect of having someone else do it to him because he is unable to help himself is quite different. The nurse must always be aware of this difference.

Caring comprises not only physical caring, but being concerned about the whole person, his feelings, fears and foibles. Respect for his needs, his privacy and wishes must be paramount in the nurse's mind. Concern also includes listening to the patient's needs and showing compassion. The nurse brings the human touch to the increasingly technological and scientific modern medical practice.

Nursing is commitment

A decision is made to become a nurse. This means commitment to accept the concepts and responsibilities that are part of nursing and include observing ethical norms and standards, concern (caring) for the person in need of care and cooperation with other members of the health team. In order to achieve this the nurse must accept responsibility for her education and training and for the maintenance of competence. She must understand and dedicate herself to the aims and objectives of the nursing profession. Commitment requires constant, conscious effort on the part of the nurse to establish a positive, clear professional self-image, an image that produces confidence and trust in those for whom she cares.

Nursing as the therapeutic use of self

The word 'therapeutic' – from the Greek *therapuein* – means to take care of, curative (Chambers 20th Century Dictionary, 4th edition). In using herself as a therapeutic agent the nurse accepts responsibility for the care of her patients/clients. She uses all her knowledge and skills, including observation of the person's condition, planning and commencing and supervising care programmes. She must take an active part in the regimen planned, supporting the person in need and his relatives and special friends.

In using herself therapeutically the professional nurse instils confidence in those for whom she is caring so that they can strive to maintain health, to regain it or to live within the limitations of ill-health. In order to achieve this the nurse herself needs confidence and self-esteem. The educational programme that prepares the nurse for practice must anticipate the needs of future practitioners and provide them with the knowledge, skills and insight necessary for making the maximum therapeutic use of self in professional practice.

MAN – THE RECIPIENT OF NURSING

In human existence nothing can be taken for granted; constant change occurs and man is continually faced with choices, decisions, and the need to adjust and adapt. Each man must live his own life, no one can do it for him, although in the living of his own life he is conscious of not only himself, but also others with whom he comes into contact. As a human being man can think, plan and determine what he feels he ought to be and ought to do.

Man is an *individual* and vested with an inner dignity. He is able to decide his own future and must make his own decisions. When in need of nursing care, a human being generally allows himself to be nursed, but the *decision to accept* nursing is still his own. Only in an unconscious or semi-conscious state may he unwittingly submit to nursing. The continued process of nursing is possible only if the nurse and the patient or client interact. However, the nurse and the other members of the health team must accept that the patient, the central human being in the action, has *freedom of choice*, that is he can accept or reject the nursing care offered.

DISRUPTION CAUSED BY ILLNESS

The patient's world is so disrupted by illness, or, in the promotive and preventive field, would be so disrupted were appropriate action not taken, that he depends on a fellow human being, in this case the nurse, to recognise his need for nursing intervention, to understand it and to listen and respond in a meaningful way to his call for help. Even the presentation of oneself for immunisation or for a routine medical examination constitutes asking for help of a specific sort from a health professional.

THE ONE WHO NURSES

So far one aspect of the nursing situation, that which concerns the person in need of nursing, has been touched upon. The other aspect of the situation concerns *the one who nurses*. By presenting herself to 'take up nursing' and thus showing her willingness to nurse, the neophyte (ie the new, usually young nursing student) commits herself to acquiring the knowledge and skills necessary to the performance of her chosen task. At the same time the *humanness* of the person in need of nursing care must be recognised. This person has his own unique characteristics which make him fundamentally different from all other human beings.

ACCEPTANCE OF THE PATIENT

The nurse must be prepared to accept the patient or client *as he is*, without judging him in any way. His feelings must be respected, especially when he is in a helpless state. The nurse helps and sustains such a person until he is able to help himself once more and develops the will to meet the future – a future which in times of illness, a crisis time in his life, may look dark, even hopeless.

A young man who has recently lost a limb in an accident is a good example of this. To him, carrying on living without a leg or an arm may seem impossible. By accepting him as he is, in his frailty and disability, the nurse may go a long way to helping him to the realisation that life may still have meaning for him, that there is a future. He thereby regains the will to live as well as his grasp on the future, and is well on the way to convalescence and rehabilitation. It is not sympathy that he needs from the nurse, but realistic acceptance, a willingness to let him express his distress and worry, and helpful, sustaining support, both physical and mental. The nurse must anticipate his needs and interpret these to other members of the health team, who often do not have such continuous contact with patients.

INDISPENSABLE ROLE OF THE NURSE

In modern society the nurse is still an indispensable person in any institution that cares for the sick, despite the enormous advances of technology. No technician, no operator of a machine, however competent, can replace the nurse. However natural and biological science-orientated her education may be, the nurse is still the one person who continuously sees the patient or client in the specific life situation in which he finds himself.

The knowledge the nurse must acquire during the course of her education includes the study of the organs of the body and their functions, as well as the pathological states that can occur and the appropriate treatment of these. She must, however, always relate this knowledge to the person in need of care, and at the same time accept him as he is, including all the disagreeable aspects that may be part of his clinical picture. A sick person, by virtue of the physical signs of illness, may be physically unattractive. This must make no difference to the attitude of the nurse offering nursing care. It is the nurse who stays with the patient, even in his weakest or incurable state. The nurse works scientifically, because she knows what she is doing and why, but in her scientific assessment of the situation and the subsequent actions based on this assessment she remains a human being who communicates with another human being in need. The nurse has many instrumental functions (ie those that are related to physical acts), but the expressive functions (ie those related to feelings, emotions and thus emotional support) remain paramount.

THE TRUST RELATIONSHIP

The sick person, or the well person who is in need of health care to keep him so, is a person in need. The nurse has special knowledge and skills and is the person to whom this need is communicated and who will be prepared to attend to that need and bring the expertise of her art and science to bear on the situation. The nurse and the sick person establish communication and a trust relationship is built up, so that the sick person is able to submit his body to the ministrations of the nurse secure in the knowledge that he will be safe in her hands, that the nurse will respect his privacy and not talk to others about his body, which is a vital part of him, in a derogatory manner, and that at all times he will be treated with respect, as a member of the human race.

All life is of equal value, irrespective of race, colour, creed, sex, age, intelligence and economic status. However, because men are individuals they can never be equal in all respects. Even uniovular twins have inequalities and differences. No two people can carry the same responsibilities to the same degree, even if they are of the same race, colour, sex, religion and age. With exactly the same opportunity, one person may be an outstanding musician and another quite hopeless at the art.

THE WORLD OF THE SICK PERSON

It is essential that the nurse realises that the world of the sick person is very different from the world of the well. The nurse, in her own uncertainty, may escape into the use of techniques and technology, leaving the sick person out of her conscious thought. The world of the sick is a disturbed and strange world to the nurse, but it is even more so to the person caught in it. His world has shrunk because of the disease or deformity that has ensnared him. The will to act is often impaired by the nature of the illness, so that the sick person now has to live with a body that will no longer carry out acts that were formerly taken for granted.

THE THREAT OF ILLNESS

Illness of a short duration may cause only a temporary cessation of normal existence, but it holds in it a latent threat. Because the experience of illness is new to him, it may be the first time that a person realises that he is mortal. He experiences, perhaps for the first time in his life, what it means not to be able to do something. It can bring with it thoughts of what it could be like not to be able to do anything ever again. The realisation of the meaning of health, of its value and importance, may bring the temporary sufferer to an understanding of the need to adopt positive measures to safeguard and preserve health once it is restored to him. Short-term, non-acute illness is usually treated at home, that is in the community. What, though, of the person whose illness is so severe that he has to be admitted to hospital because he needs specific medical or surgical intervention? His life world is now drastically changed. His independence is affected. He is powerless to help himself. He leaves his home and his work environment, where he is known, where he has enjoyed a certain status, has had responsibilities, and has participated in the decision making of others, as well as having made his own plans. This chain of events is broken. He may even be carried out of his home or from his work situation and conveyed to hospital in an ambulance. He is now in the hands of others, dependent where once he regulated his own life.

DANGER OF DEPERSONALISATION

On entry to hospital the situation may even worsen. Cold officialdom may take over. He must furnish all kinds of information about his affairs, which formerly were of concern only to him and perhaps to his nearest and dearest. These penetrating questions are asked by complete strangers. He is no longer an individual, but is placed in a file, on a chart. A part of his being has become an official document and he feels anonymous. He is then pushed away to another part of the building, to an X-ray department or to a ward, where another stranger receives him and puts him to bed and where he is perhaps required to give up his clothes. Another part of him is thus removed. It is now possible that he will be washed by yet another stranger and his body is looked upon by that stranger – something quite outside his previous experience. He loses part of himself each time. If care is not taken, the officialdom of the hospital can reduce the human being to an object, depersonalise him.

AVAILABILITY OF THE NURSE

The thinking, caring nurse should be available at all stages of this process through the efficient machine that is the modern hospital. She is the one who, understanding the needs of the human being, helps and sustains him through these assaults on his life world. Nursing, by its very nature, helps the sick person, the vulnerable human being, to come to terms with his illness, to accept the help of strangers in this place where he would much rather not be, if he had any real choice. The nurse must also realise that the world of the person condemned to chronic sickness or deformity is so radically changed that this person is in great need of support of a very special kind if he is to find meaning in life once more and to look forward to the future with anticipation of further interesting days.

VARIOUS DEFINITIONS

Nursing has been defined by many people in different ways, according to individual background and philosophy. The definition at which the writer has arrived for herself may be expressed as follows:

> Nursing is that service to mankind which enables people to attain and maintain good health and to prevent illness, or, when illness occurs, helps and supports them, so that they may overcome their illness and regain full health. If this ideal of complete restoration to health is unattainable (man, after all, is mortal), then nursing should help and support the person to make the maximum use of any potential left. In the last resort, nursing should sustain the person and his family, so that he may die in peace and with dignity.

The South African Nursing Council has recently defined nursing as follows:

> Nursing science is a human clinical science that constitutes the body of knowledge for the practice of persons registered or enrolled under the Nursing Act, as nurses or midwives. Within the parameters of nursing philosophy and ethics, it is concerned with the development of knowledge for the nursing diagnosis, treatment and personalised health care of persons exposed to or suffering or recovering from physical or mental ill-health. It encompasses the study of preventive, promotive, curative and rehabilitative health care for individuals, for families, groups and communities and covers man's life-span from before birth.

Charlotte Searle, in her inaugural lecture as professor of nursing at the University of Pretoria (Credo, Unisa guide NUE 003/1, pp. 3, 4), said that nursing can fulfil its allotted task only if it has an intellectual, philosophical and disciplined approach to man's health needs. She saw the philosophical landmarks of nursing as follows:

- The *belief* in the essential *meaning* and *worth* of every human life
- The *recognition* of the *uniqueness* of every human life
- The *responsibility* that the Creator has placed in the hands of man for the welfare of his fellow-man
- *Trust* that there will always be an inner strength that will enable one to cope and help one to make the right decision
- A *yearning* to be a worthy servant of mankind and of medical science
- *Acceptance* of the fact that nursing has instrumental and expressive dimensions and that it is not disease that matters, but patients who are ill and threatened
- *Overcoming* a tendency toward a nurse/patient relationship in favour of the relationship between one human being and another and an overcoming of all obstacles in the provision of health care
- *Change and conservation* – conservation of a precious human life and assistance to those who are vulnerable through change. All nursing is aimed at prevention, promotion, change, balance and conservation

- ☐ *Help and support*, not only to those in need of health care but also to fellow workers
- ☐ Development of a nursing *technology* in the application of scientific principles, knowledge and skills
- ☐ The therapeutic use of self.

Thus nursing cares for people in need of a specific type of care, and is based on respect for the human being coupled with knowledge and skills acquired over a long period of education. Additions are made to this knowledge and skill throughout the professional lives of the practitioners of nursing.

SYMBOLISM OF THE LAMP

Traditionally nurses light a lamp and take a pledge of service on their entry into the professional ranks. The symbolism of the lamp is often missed, although the lamp has a very special significance in the philosophy of the nursing profession.

The lamp symbolises that the nurse must be the light along the path of those who are experiencing dark and difficult days as a result of breakdowns in health, or who have a need for special insight into their health problems or the prevention of such problems. Nursing, by its very nature, offers a beacon of light, metaphorically at least, to those who need help in their pain and suffering, to those who need someone to do for them what they are unable to do for themselves. Persons in need of health care and those near and dear to them need the constant help and support of the nurse when they face discomfort, severe pain or actual or impending death. The trust relationship that is built up, the nurse's approachability, her *being there*, in person, is a beacon of light to those going through a crisis in health, indeed in having life as they know it. This occurs in the community as well as the hospital setting.

The nursing profession, through its members the nurses, must be a light to mankind during any crisis situation related to health. Many crises which have health implications arise in everyday life. Nurses are trained to deal with crises affecting health. The technical skill and empathetic handling of these crises is also symbolised by the light of the lamp.

The lamp symbolises a pledge to give service with human understanding to those who need it; that the nurse, as an individual, will be a light of hope to the unique person to whom care is given in the course of nursing practice.

The lamp also stands for the light of knowledge and science that is fundamental to the practice of nursing. The light of knowledge must not be allowed to become dim, it must be kept alive by practice, reading, updating, research, continuing to learn and to grow as a professional. The lamp also stands for the light of faith, faith in religious principles, faith in what the nurse is doing and faith in the meaning of life. The light of faith underlines the caring profession of nursing.

If the nurse approaches her task in the light of this background she will become a true nurse, a full professional practitioner.

THEORIES OF NURSING

Many people have sought to describe a theory of nursing, but to date there has been a great difference of opinion and no clear theory has crystallised.

A theory is an explanation of a system or of the abstract principles of a science or art.

Imogen King, in her book *Toward a theory of Nursing* (1971), attempted 'to explore dimensions of nursing and to propose a conceptual frame of reference for professional nursing'. She states that 'this book has departed from previous attempts by nurses to formulate theoretical approaches for nursing' (King 1971: 2).

Martha Rogers, Jeanne Quint, Virginia S Cleland, Irene Brown, Hildegard Peplau and others have all tackled the subject from different points of view, while more recent writers such as Marjorie Gordon, Myra Levine, Dorothy Johnson, Dorothy Orem, Callista Roy, Zderad and Paterson, and others are not yet in agreement on the subject. It is unnecessary for a basic student to study this aspect in any detail. She must just be aware that people are interested in the subject and are trying to arrive at a satisfactory point of departure for those practising clinical nursing, nurse philosophers, nurse educators and others. More advanced students would do well to obtain and read what these and other prominent nurse leaders have to say and keep up to date with developing or evolving patterns of thought.

Holistic nursing is a term that appears frequently in nursing literature today. Myra Levine, a great protagonist of this approach, says 'the holistic approach to nursing can depend on the recognition of the integrated response of the individual arising from the internal environment and the interaction which occurs with the external environment'. Further she believes that *all nursing is 'conservation' or keeping together*, and that the nurse, by balancing nursing action and patient participation within the safe limits of the patient's ability to participate in his care, can help to restore 'wholeness' in his health situation while respecting his dignity, his privacy and his right to retain his independence. The nurse helps the patient to find security and balance in the environment in which he finds himself and in which he must live (extract from a paper presented at the Nurse Educator Conference in New York in 1978).

2 Evolution of nursing: historical trends

ETHOS – THE CHARACTER AND NATURE

The ethos of nursing is concerned with the character or nature of nursing. This has not come into being out of a vacuum, but has been formed by its historical development. Nursing history, however, is part of the mainstream of history and not something separate.

As changes have occurred in the history of the world diverse health patterns have developed. Health care delivery systems have evolved to meet the need that has arisen due to man's environment to provide not only for survival, but also for prosperity. Many of the changes wrought by man have brought with them unforeseen health hazards, for example pollution of the air which followed the introduction of technology in the form of factories. Fortunately, man's ingenuity has found the answer to this particular dilemma, but as one hazard is conquered another crops up. Without this evolution much of the excitement that keeps man alert and future orientated would be lost, to the detriment of his existence as a human being.

History is exciting

The study of nursing history should present an adventure to all who are engaged in it. Everyone in this life has an interest in the past, for the past has brought us to where we are. The past also points the way to the future, so that we can avoid the pitfalls of the days that are behind. We can look to what lies ahead, secure in the knowledge that problems in the past, insurmountable as they may have seemed at the time, were overcome. This should give us the courage to tackle any special difficulties as and when they occur.

Many excellent books on the history of nursing are recommended for detailed study; particularly those dealing with the evolution of nursing through the ages and which discern the historical trends that have shaped nursing.

This chapter will look at certain aspects of nursing history particularly as they affect the nursing scene in the Republic of South Africa. It should be read in conjunction with other books on nursing history and general history, and not instead of them.

The first chapter attempted to clarify the nature of nursing. Here the intention is to highlight certain occurrences in general history and in the development of other professions and to point out the relationship between these occurrences and the development of nursing as it is known today.

The reader will be able to gain insight into the trends in the past that made the present and lead to the future. History is around us. We are today writing the history that will be studied tomorrow.

THE EFFECT OF VARIOUS FACTORS ON THE EVOLUTION OF NURSING

Religion

All men, thoughout recorded history, have held some belief in a power outside themselves, a supreme being or beings. This has varied from belief in the 'magical powers' of inanimate objects, totem poles, amulets, statues and the like to ancestor worship and belief in the existence of intangible beings, spirits or gods who had the fate of men in their powers. 'Religious' belief or belief in supernatural powers developed into 'systems of faith' or 'religions'. In one form or another these religions have influenced man's life, his work, his attitudes and his relationships. This means that they have had an influence on nursing, which affects all men.

Primitive cultures found the causes of disease difficult to understand. A cut from a sharp stone and its damage to the body was visible, and therefore clear, but there appeared to be no logical explanation for internal pain, vomiting, coughing, fever and paralysis. Empirical remedies were found by trial and error, but the use of these treatments was often combined with 'magic' practices.

Origin of medicine

Medical practice has its origins in the belief that magic could cure or prevent ill-health. The powers of magic were thought to be embodied in the persons of shamans or witch-doctors. Evil spirits, which appeared to be attacking people and causing the inexplicable symptoms of disease, had to be placated and encouraged to leave the bodies of the afflicted or warded off. The shamans developed ritualistic practices as part of their method of treatment.

At the same time ancestor worship prevented the study of the dead human body. This held up the development of medical knowledge and thus of nursing. In Ancient China, for example, medical knowledge was limited to the use of herbal remedies, knowledge that was entirely empirical. Massage, which was also practised, may have developed from punishing the body to drive out the evil spirits.

Temples – Priest-physicians

As societies became more sophisticated the worshipping of one of the gods accepted in an area became concentrated in one specific place. Those who were ill came to the place of worship of the god in whom they believed in order to get the priests of that system of worship (religion) to pray for a cure, or to help them to pacify the gods. A fixed community grew up in that area and a temple for the worship of that particular god was built. In charge of the temples were priests who, because they also helped to treat the sick, became known as priest-physicians. Many sick people stayed at the temples for 'treatment' and temple attendants looked after them. Perhaps these were the first nurses, other than the mothers and other members of the family who, until then, had cared for the sick, injured and helpless.

The effects of some widespread religions are discussed briefly below.

Buddhism

This religion had its origins in the sixth century BCE with an Indian prince, *Siddhartha Guatama*, who became known as the 'Enlightened One'. Buddhism spread rapidly throughout India and to Burma, Ceylon, Thailand, China, Mongolia, Korea and Japan. It even reached the Tatars of South Eastern Russia (*World of Knowledge Encyclopaedia*). Buddhism states that pain and suffering exist and that man is doomed to suffer. As long as man strives for himself and for the pleasures of this life, he will suffer. This interest in his own good and striving for the good things in life must be overcome before pain and suffering can be conquered.

Because of this teaching disease was thought to be caused by straying from the correct course set for man to gain enlightenment, and was therefore a just punishment which had to be endured. This belief was not conducive to the development of medical knowledge or of nursing.

In later times Buddhism largely disappeared from India, to be replaced by Hinduism. It still flourishes in other parts of the world.

Hinduism

This is a comprehensive term used to designate the social customs and religious beliefs of the majority of people in present-day India.

Hinduism developed in India between the fifth and fourth centuries BCE. It has many different important gods, including Brahma, Shiva, Vishnu and Krishna. Brahma is the supreme being in the Hindu pantheon, many other gods being seen as manifestations of him. Brahma cannot be clearly delineated.

The Brahman 'scriptures or writings', the *Vedas*, were believed to be a divine gift from Brahma. These books were the historical documents of India and their doctrines were presented in the form of hymns, prayers and teachings (Donahue 1985: 59). The *Vedas* and commentaries on them discussed, *inter alia*, the medicinal use of herbs and the use of incantations to treat physical ills. Because these were 'sacred' books, the religious aspects of Hindu 'medical' practice are obvious.

The Hebrew religion

Hebrews were monotheistic, worshipping only one god. The high priests of this religion practised as priest-physicians and health inspectors, basing their practices on the Mosaic Code, the law given to Moses by God.

This 'law' was an organised set of rules for the prevention of disease and the promotion of health. It included aspects of personal hygiene, female hygiene in relation to menstruation and childbirth, the slaughtering of animals for food, the disposal of refuse and human excreta and control of communicable diseases, including recognition, isolation, quarantine and disinfection. Again this was a 'divine order' and the religious rules affected health care in a broad sense.

The religion of the Ancient Greeks

The ancient Greeks developed a special god of healing, Apollo, whose son Asklepios was the God of Medicine. Hygeia, the goddess of health, and Panacea, the goddess of medication, were daughters of Asklepios. A large temple dedicated to Asklepios was built at Epidauros and a medical centre grew up around the temple.

Hippocrates, generally known as the 'father of medicine', belonged to an Asklepiad family. The Asklepiades were an order of priests who were supposed to be descended from Asklepios and claimed a knowledge of medicine.

The Hippocratic Oath, which set a standard for medical ethics, commenced with the words 'I swear by Apollo, the healer, by Asklepios, by health and all the powers of healing, and call to witness all the gods and goddesses that I may keep this oath . . .'. It was used to initiate men into the art and practice of medicine. Again the practice of medicine was clearly linked with religion (see Appendix A).

Christianity

This religion exerted a great influence on health care – Christianity was largely concerned with the recognition of every man's human worth as an individual. Service to man was service to God.

Nursing as a separate entity began in the early Christian period. Before this time the care of the sick, except by those nearest and dearest to them, was entrusted to slaves. Christian service to the sick spread into the community; orders of deaconesses and monastic orders were established, and the nuns 'who took the veil' started an influence on nursing and nursing history that has endured to this day.

The Emperor Julian (c 331-363) stated that the care given by Christians to the sick was one of the factors that made them enemies of the then powerful Roman gods.

The Protestant revolution, a religious movement in Christianity, initially did a great deal of harm to medicine and nursing because of the destruction of monastries and convents and their attached hospitals. The revival of the deaconess orders by the Protestant churches led to a renewed awareness of the care of the sick as a religious duty and missions to all parts of the world opened up health care to many people as hospitals developed alongside evangelism. In Southern Africa it was the Christian missions that paved the way for the training of Black women as nurses.

Florence Nightingale saw her work among the sick as a Christian duty. Sister Henrietta Stockdale of the Anglican Sisterhood of St Michael and All Angels and other sisters of that order had a profound effect on the formal training of nurses in South Africa and on the introduction of state registration in the Cape in 1891, the first state registration of nurses in the world.

When studying nursing history in more detail students can trace the effects of religions on health care and thus on nursing. Other religious beliefs can be reviewed to see what influences they may have had on health care. Many more instances of the effects of religions on the development of nursing can be found. What has been incorporated here is meant to serve only as a guide to the concept of religious influence on nursing.

Wars

From the earliest times men have waged war on one another, but it is not only the effects of the weapons used by both sides to kill the enemy that have influenced medicine and nursing. Many armies have been defeated and the course of history changed by the *occurrence of epidemic diseases* following on the disruption of sanitary and hygiene practices and the breakdown of order. Bubonic plague and other epidemic diseases often became rampant. Many more soldiers were killed by disease than by enemy action.

In the earliest times slaves looked after the sick and wounded combatants during war. The Romans erected large, well-planned hospitals for the men in the army. The sick and wounded in these hospitals were tended by military personnel as well as by slaves.

The Crusades, which were religious wars waged in an attempt to wrest the Holy Land from the infidel, resulted in the formation of well-organised military nursing orders to look after Crusaders. Their objectives were religious as much as military, so that a combination of religious and military influence is seen in the nursing services that developed. These military nursing orders included The Knights Hospitallers of St John of Jerusalem, the Knights of St Lazarus, and the Teutonic Knights. The orders built some fine hospitals and in them good hospital administration practices were developed and carried out. Although instituted to care for the sick and wounded soldiers fighting in the Crusades, these orders also cared for all who participated in pilgrimages to the Holy Land.

Many nursing traditions which are still honoured today have their origins in military nursing, which dates back to the Crusades. These include the rigid etiquette that was followed by military orders, the rounds with the physicians and the physical pattern of nursing units, with a large ward for the less ill patients, side wards for the more seriously ill and cubicles for those in a critical state.

Despite these early developments resulting in the establishment of military nursing orders, military medicine, which aimed at treating sick as well as wounded soldiers, was slow to develop. It was only at the end of the eighteenth century that military medicine became part of the organisation of the army and a permanent medical corps, army hospitals and field medical casualty stations became a reality.

The Napoleonic wars finally brought disaster to the French nation, which lost large numbers of its force through disease. This event brought France to the realisation that there was a great need for really efficient medical care for soldiers during war time. The Crimean War did the same for the British when Florence Nightingale, working with a heterogeneous group of Catholic nuns, Anglican sisters and lay nurses, brought the death rate of those treated in Scutari down from 427 to 22 per thousand. This she achieved by sanitary reforms, serving proper diets, training orderlies and proper individual care. She fought a bitter battle to achieve these reforms and eventually established nursing as a respectable profession for which training was necessary.

The Crimean War and the experience Florence Nightingale gained because of it has moulded the pattern of modern nursing in no uncertain way. The American Civil War was another national disaster in which twice as many soldiers succumbed to disease as to battle wounds.

International Red Cross

Another tremendous influence on the care of sick and wounded soldiers was that exercised by *Henri Dunant*, who, by chance, stumbled on to the battlefield of Solferino after the battle between the armies of Napoleon III and Austria in 1859. He was so upset by the sufferings of the wounded and dying that he attempted to bring some order into the chaos and to organise nearby villagers to give some form of care to the wounded. This experience was such a nightmare that he wrote an article *'Un Souvenir de Solferino'* (1862) in which he proposed a plan for dealing with any such future event. This plan involved international cooperation and his writings and efforts led eventually to the foundation, in 1863, of the International Committee of the Red Cross at the Geneva Convention.

This is the greatest humanitarian movement that the world has even known. Today the Red Cross societies of various nations, united under the International Committee, not only care for those suffering as a result of wars, but provide or coordinate aid for people affected by any disaster. Thus relief is given to those in need as a result of floods, famine, earthquakes and other such occurrences.

The nurse in the military nursing services performs an important role. Her traditional role of providing nursing services to all people, irrespective of race, colour or creed, friend or enemy, is entrenched in the Geneva Convention.

However, the military nursing orders, the military medical and nursing service and the formation of the Red Cross are not entirely responsible for alleviating the lot of the soldier. Advances in preventive medicine, with the resultant immunisation and standards of sanitation, have also played a large part. In the past the nurse has played a very important part in improving the health care of army personnel and will continue to do so in the future.

Exploration and colonisation

From very early times men have tended to move away from their place of birth and 'discover' other parts of the world. This tendency was strengthened by the European countries seeking a sea route to the East, 'discovering' Africa and its peoples, 'discovering' the 'New World' (the Americas) and eventually colonising great continents. The 'voyages of discovery' themselves were subject to many health hazards, not the least of which was scurvy.

The contact that the early settlers had with the indigenous peoples of the lands in which they settled had definite health implications for both groups. There was fighting, which brought its own miseries. The settlers came into contact with tropical diseases that were new to them and climates with which they were unfamiliar. The indigenous people, on the other hand, through contact with the settlers were exposed to infectious diseases that they had not encountered before and many indigenous populations were decimated by diseases such as measles and smallpox because they had no inbuilt resistance to them.

On the credit side, colonisation brought with it health care of a more sophisticated nature from the colonising power. The type of care varied with the stage of development of health care attained by the country that 'exported' its system of health care.

The activities of missionaries often preceded formal colonisation and continued when an area was colonised, contributing greatly to the development of health care systems in the new settlements.

In the process of exporting Western cultural patterns the colonising powers attempted to educate the people native to the colonised land, and with general education went education of health personnel to meet the needs of the times.

Social change

Social change is any change that occurs in the structure of society. It is a neutral concept implying neither progression nor regression, although it may be either. Social change occurs in every society and has done so since the beginning of man's history, but it is not necessarily similar in each society. It may occur gradually, by evolution, or in some cases by revolution.

Nursing has developed as a subsystem of society and as such has changed and evolved in response to changing social needs. Health care needs have altered throughout history as a result of various factors such as new habits and customs which alter disease patterns, migration and the grouping together of people in large numbers for protection, for the production of food or some other commodity, or for recreation.

Whether regressive or progressive social change is continuous. The factors that influence social change are dealt with below.

Environmental factors

The physical or geographical environment of man (including the soil, the geographical situation in which he finds himself, the climate and natural resources) contributes to social change. The physical environment may be restrictive when arid land is inhabited or it may be promotive where there is an abundance of water and other natural resources.

Man, by his very nature, can and does make changes in his physical environment which enable him to survive and often thrive in an adverse physical environment. He can tame nature by the use of scientific agricultural methods, the draining of marshes, the building of dams and the institution of irrigation schemes. He has been able to create an artificial environment in order to venture beyond this planet. He can survive for long periods, with suitable equipment, under the sea.

The effect on health of these changes in the physical environment must not be forgotten. The draining of the Italian marshes led to the eradication of the malarial mosquito in that area. Space medicine has opened up new vistas in the treatment of human disease which had their origins in man's need to create an environment in which he could travel to outer space. The new knowledge gained of human physiology was a bonus resulting from an environmental need. The achievement of a suitable environment in which a population can grow up and enjoy good health is a constant aim of Community Health Authorities. Modern sanitation is a result of man's ingenuity in changing his environment. He can also pollute it, and does so, thus being the cause of health hazards which need further attention and care in the environmental context.

Population factors

The increase or decrease in a population due to birth, birth control and death plays an important part in social change. The over-population of an area can lead to the exhaustion of its food resources, poverty, malnutrition and general ill-health. Because of her intimate association with all phases of human life, the nurse can play a significant role in social change due to population factors. Her role in family planning services is a case in point.

Urbanisation

Linked with the mechanisation of agriculture depopulation of the platteland has occurred, with a concomitant increase in urbanisation. The implications of this social change due to population factors are important in the health field.

Attitudes to health care

Attitudes to disease and suffering are influenced by custom, by religious teaching and by the values and norms upon which moral principles pertaining in a particular society are based. Increased wealth in a country does not necessarily increase health unless it is properly distributed and properly used.

Changes in living and sanitary practices are also necessary. Knowledge alone also does not provide health for all.

Today man knows what is necessary for a healthy lifestyle, yet he continues to neglect health practices. Man knows how to prevent many diseases and yet at least half of the population of the world continues to perish from these diseases. Underdeveloped countries have access to the knowledge of disease prevention. However, their own stage of development and rate of social change preclude its use.

Need for trained manpower

Trained manpower should be available. If social change has not yet produced enough educated people to undertake medical, nursing and paramedical training, then the type of health service and how it is organised will be affected. Nursing in specific areas also depends on this aspect of social change. The economy of the country is inevitably linked with this lack or otherwise of trained health service personnel.

Demographic changes in society are also related to the type of service, medical and nursing, that is necessary and that will influence the categories and areas of specialisation of medical and nursing personnel and their preparation.

Attitude to human life

The attitude of society towards human life and its sanctity is also important. Where life as such is little valued, measures to ensure its preservation are also of little interest. Changes in society's values are all that can alter this. Despite all the logical arguments that can be advanced for family planning, major changes in social attitudes are necessary to make a success of such a campaign in a social group where large families are socially valued.

History is really the story of social change throughout the ages. As health needs have changed, so medicine and nursing have developed to meet these needs. As knowledge has been broadened, social change has followed. One has only to consider any specific social change that has occurred in history to be able to trace the concomitant trends in nursing history. Change brings with it challenges. Nursing history has met these challenges in the past and will continue to do so in the future.

The status of women

The status of women in various communities, in different countries and at various times in history has affected the development of nursing and the type of nurse that has emerged. When women have been assigned low status in the community nursing has not achieved the same recognition, nor has it developed to the same extent as an independent profession, as it has in countries or communities where women have a high social status.

The need for education

In order to acquire the knowledge and skills of a highly competent, well-prepared professional person, a person must have a certain standard of basic education. In areas where the status of women in society is low their access to the higher levels of basic education is restricted and thus it is difficult, if not impossible, to train skilled nursing practitioners who are able to meet highly sophisticated health care needs. The larger number of male nurses in some societies bears this out. Although nursing worldwide has been a predominantly female profession, in some countries men have had to take a greater place in nursing practice because their general education has made it possible for them to be educated as professional nurses, training which is denied their lesser-educated sisters.

The high status in society of women like Florence Nightingale at a time in nursing history when, apart from that given by the religious sisterhoods, nursing was carried out by women of the lower classes, women of questionable character who were promiscuous and troublesome and had an inordinate thirst for alcoholic beverages and other unmentionable vices, gave nursing a respectability which helped it to evolve from its dark ages (Woodham-Smith 1951: 47, 48, 108).

The emancipation of women

The movement that brought about the emancipation of women in the western world eventually changed the status of women, and thus also of nurses, and led to tremendous developments in nursing knowledge and skills and in the art and science of nursing.

In a multinational land where the status of women in various cultural groups is different, the availability of enough women with an educational background sufficient to allow them to train as professional nurses has in the past presented problems which are steadily being overcome.

Global picture of nursing

In their study of the ethos of nursing it is important that nurses have a global picture of all aspects affecting nursing. The status of women in society is one of the determinants of the characteristics of nursing in that society and thus is part of the ethos of nursing, concerned, as it is, with the evolution, the development and the expansion of nursing, past, present and future.

Scientific and technological developments

The effects of religion, wars and social change have already received consideration. Two of the factors that have markedly affected nursing are the rapid advance in the knowledge available to the natural and biological scientist and the technology that has grown out of this over the last few decades.

In the study of the ethos of nursing we are concerned with the implications of various trends in the disciplines involved in the field of health care.

Science and technology have armed medicine with so many revolutionary technological devices and scientific discoveries that medical practice and therefore nursing, which is a basic component of medicine, has changed dramatically. If, as sociologists tell us, there have been greater advances in medicine in the almost seven decades of the twentieth century than in all the decades since Hippocrates of Cos (460-359 BCE), then the tremendous impact on the lives of people and those who serve them in the health team must be obvious.

The first scientist

Thales of Miletus, a Greek philosopher who lived between 636 and 546 BCE, is generally regarded as the founder of abstract geometry and the earliest Greek scientist – in fact the first scientist.

During the ages scientific discovery and scientific knowledge gradually increased. In the seventeenth century a paradoxical situation occurred when the knowledge acquired by natural scientists developed over a broad spectrum of activity but medical knowledge remained static, in fact some was lost so that the sum total was actually less. The great progress in anatomical knowledge during the second half of the sixteenth century had very little effect on the surgery performed during the seventeenth century. Many misconceptions were incorporated in what was in any case minimal knowledge. There has been a remarkable change during the present century. It has been stated that there are as many scientists alive today as the total number who had lived up to the beginning of the century. As scientific knowledge advanced rapidly, and with it technology, scientific training for nurses became an urgent necessity if they were to be able to play their part in the scientific world of modern medicine.

Need for scientific background

As early as 1797 Dr Franz May of Mannheim, Germany, said that poor nursing due to a lack of scientific training was an important cause of hospital deaths (Searle 1965: ch 10). It was because of this lack that he started a nurse training school at Heidelberg University. This school preceded the Nightingale school by more than 50 years.

Lord Lister, generally regarded as the father of antiseptic surgery, lived from 1827 to 1912. His work with carbolic acid started in 1865, the latter half of the nineteenth century. Surgical aseptic technique, which replaced Lister's technique, is therefore a very late technological development. The use of rubber gloves by surgeons and nurses was introduced by William Halstead in 1890. Constant improvements in sterilising techniques continue to this day.

The incredible advances that have been made in the fields of medicine and surgery owe much of their development to technology and to scientific inquiry. These advances are common knowledge much publicised in the popular press. There are new techniques, new instruments and new drugs, all of which appear with such frequency that it is well-nigh impossible to remain conversant with what is happening around one. One has only to think of dialysis machines, heart-lung machines, monitors, respirators, defibrillators, antibiotics and the drugs used to control mental illness to get an idea of what scientific and technological development has meant to the health care delivery system.

It has been estimated that major medical advances occurred at the rate of about one every century up to 1900. After that the number of important discoveries affecting medical care suddenly increased to about one every ten years until 1940. Thereafter the tempo increased to about one new development per year and today new developments are possibly even more frequent. Ninety percent of the drugs used routinely today were unknown a decade ago.

Constant advances are being made in diagnostic techniques and in the treatment of cardiovascular and metabolic diseases and malignancies. Genetic conditions are recognisable before birth. Nuclear energy is being harnessed for good as well as for evil. Safe oral contraception is commonplace. Will the menopause also be delayed? Certain communicable diseases have been eradicated. Despite these advances, new problems constantly rear their heads.

The effects of scientific and technological developments on medicine and on nursing are easily discernible. With all the aids at man's disposal early detection of disease conditions becomes possible and subsequent treatment keeps people active in society for much longer. The promotive and preventive aspects of disease management have come into their own and offer exciting challenges to the nurses of today and tomorrow. The scientific revolution that has occurred in medicine has brought about an intricate interrelationship between medical men, research laboratories, techniques, pharmacologists, chemists, computer scientists, engineers and many more.

No longer do the doctor, nurse and pharmacist assume responsibility for the total care of the patient. We now have electronic and nuclear aids for diagnosis and treatment, organ transplants, cardiac catheterisation and immuno-suppressive drugs. Diseases, diagnoses and treatments that were little understood or unknown half a century ago are commonplace today. Space medicine is with us. Nurses take part in the relevant research programmes.

Medical science has overcome many diseases, but as a result of the creation of a longer life span the number of people subject to chronic and geriatric diseases has escalated. Iatrogenic diseases, which create new problems, are rapidly increasing. Nursing will also develop more and more along specialist lines, but within the body of the art is the science of nursing as a whole; the renal care nurse, the intensive care nurse, with perhaps even more specialisation into the realms of pulmonary or cardiovascular subdivisions, and neurological nurse specialists are examples.

Scientific and technological development have made all these possible. The preparation of the nurse to meet these challenges must obviously also take on new dimensions. The time has come for all professional nurse educators to keep their goals, curricula and facilities under careful and continuous review so that their students are equipped to meet the revolutionary changes that are occurring around them in their spheres of work. Not only must they be ready for changes, but they must participate in research and innovate techniques of their own.

Medical science has developed extensively during the past decades. The ratio of medical practitioners to the population and to other members of the health team varies considerably. The more remote areas are generally not well supplied with medical men, who tend to congregate in cities. This tendency puts a greater burden on other members of the team, in particular the nurse. The numbers of nurses of all categories available to serve the community, even in remote areas, have made it possible for health services to be instituted or expanded where before no service, or only a limited service, was possible. Nurses' technological skills have had to be increased to meet the needs for these services.

Evolving role of the nurse

Nursing has evolved and, because it is a dynamic profession, is still evolving and will continue to do so. It has become fashionable today to talk of the 'expanded' or the 'extended' role of the nurse as though this is a new concept. Perhaps the role of the nurse has evolved more rapidly in the past few decades than ever before in history, but this is only in line with the development of medical and scientific knowledge and practice. More and more specialisation has occurred in medicine and in nursing.

The nurse and the doctor, because of their interdependence, have come to realise that there is no absolute demarcation between their functions. The doctor, because of his training, is the leader of the medical team, both legally and in practice. However, due to the thin spread of medical practitioners, his role is evolving into one of being on tap and not on top.

The difference between the functions of doctors and nurses is one of depth and range. Both have instrumental and expressive functions.

Modern medicine must be made available to the patient, but the developments in medicine have made it more and more difficult for the doctor to maintain close personal contact with patients. He has to devote a great deal of time to keeping abreast of the new technology of medicine and to consulting with specialists and other members of the health team. The doctor's role has evolved — so has that of the nurse. This is a natural development of the process of evolution.

The role of the professional nurse must of necessity change alongside those of the other health professionals. Her knowledge and skills must be developed and broadened. She must be prepared to accept more responsibilities in the future if the needs of the clients of modern sophisticated medicine are to be fully met. She must not only receive adequate educational preparation to enable her to accept this role, but must also be shown that her role is innovative and constantly evolving. She must think, investigate, plan, implement and evaluate throughout her professional life. Just as in the past the nurse took over the role which until that time had been exclusively the prerogative of the physician, so she must relinquish some of her present-day techniques to lesser-qualified persons, the semi-professional groups of nurses (enrolled) and nurses' assistants, as she moves into hitherto unknown fields.

At the same time the professional nurse must be careful to maintain her concern with the patient as a person – her *caring* function cannot be withdrawn if she is still to be worthy of the name nurse. Nursing must not be allowed to evolve in a direction that leaves caring to others. On the contrary, the modern future nurse will *exercise her care with more understanding of the human being and in greater depth* than ever before. Her role has evolved in the realm of primary care and must do so more in the future.

Primary care can be seen as the person's *first contact* with any member of the health team. Such contact can be made to prevent illness, to promote health or to obtain assistance at the onset of any given episode of illness, often seeking assistance for the first time.

In many instances this first contact is made with the nurse, who must be prepared to undertake tasks currently required, such as:

☐ routine assessment of the health status of patients and families
☐ taking and recording a health history
☐ assessing deviations from normal in patients presenting for treatment, screening and referring
☐ evaluating the progress of treatment, for reference when necessary
☐ interpreting laboratory findings
☐ initiating therapy in minor ailments and in emergencies such as haemorrhage, cardiac arrest, pulmonary arrest, shock, poisoning, etc
☐ assessing the environment as it affects the health of the individual or family
☐ assessing community resources and their availability, means of reference, etc
☐ conducting nursing clinics.

Nursing is concerned with the total care of the patient and has a coordinating role in ensuring this type of care from all members of the health team. Thus the management function of the nurse must also receive attention. Evolving roles require evolving education in a dynamic profession.

CONTRIBUTION OF VARIOUS GROUPS TO THE EVOLUTION OF NURSING IN SOUTH AFRICA

When considering the ethos of nursing it is necessary to look at factors that may have affected its development and to try to identify factors that will affect its future.

As in other parts of the world, the development of nursing in South Africa has been influenced by many factors. South Africa has been the subject of 'discovery' by European nations – the Portuguese in the persons of Bartolomeu Dias (1488) and Vasco Da Gama (1497) rounded the Cape in search of a sea route to India. It is believed that many centuries before the Phoenicians circumnavigated the Cape, establishing temporary settlements en route. The first hospital on the Southern African continent was erected in Mozambique.

Because of its history Central and Southern Africa, as a colonised area of the world, was subjected to various influences by different European nations such as the Portuguese in Mozambique and Angola, the French in the Congo (French) and part of Cameroun, the Belgians in the Belgian Congo, the British in Rhodesia and Nyasaland (Zambia, Zimbabwe, Malawi), Bechuanaland (Botswana), Basutoland (Lesotho), Swaziland, Kenya, etc as well as the Union of South Africa, the Germans in South West Africa (Namibia) and Tanganyika (now part of Tanzania), and others.

The Southern African region was subjected to epidemics, wars and other health hazards. The contribution of various important groups to the development of nursing in South Africa will be presented in an abridged form.

The Dutch

The area that became the Union and then the Republic of South Africa was first settled by the Dutch (The Dutch East India Company) to serve as a halfway house between Holland and Batavia providing ships with fresh water and food.

In April 1652 Jan van Riebeeck brought the first band of proper settlers to Southern Africa. Thus the colonisation of the Cape took place because of a health need of sailors. A temporary hospital was built in 1656. The Dutch occupied the Cape for 143 years. Hospital care was not very good, but the Dutch brought with them their excellent pattern of midwifery (Searle 1965: chs 11, 12 and 13).

The British

The first British occupation of the Cape lasted from 1795 to 1803. When the Batavian authorities regained control in 1803 there were only 70 to 80 British settlers among the White population numbering some 30 000.

The first British occupation had little effect on health care practices, but a change took place after the reoccupation of the Cape by the British in 1807. The Supreme Medical Committee was established in 1807 and was to have far-reaching effects on both the medical and the nursing services.

The first civilian hospital

The first civilian hospital was established in Cape Town in 1818 by Dr Samuel Bailey and was known as Bailey's Somerset Hospital. Eventually rules which actually contained the seeds of a code of ethical behaviour for nurses were drawn up for the control of the hospital. These rules also contained the first principles of organisation to be applied to the running of civilian hospitals in South Africa (Searle 1965: chs 5 and 6).

The 1820 Settlers

British settlement in the Eastern Cape was reinforced by the arrival of the 1820 Settlers. These first 4 000 settlers (1 455 men, 795 women and 1 750 children) arrived in Algoa Bay as part of an assisted emigration scheme from Britain. The 1820 Settlers and others who came soon after were settled in border areas between existing White settlements and the Black tribes.

Despite the dangers and difficulties that faced them they made a tremendous contribution to the development of medical and nursing care in the area in which they settled, and later in the whole of the Cape. The military medical men, who were of a high calibre, were attached to border regiments and made a tremendous contribution to the development of hospitals in the 'frontier' or border areas. It is interesting to note that the Provincial Hospital, Port Elizabeth, was established in 1856, the Albany Hospital in Grahamstown in 1858 and the Frontier Hospital, Queenstown, in 1876. In 1874 the Board of the Provincial Hospital in Port Elizabeth obtained the services of two professionally trained nurses from England who were the first trained and qualified nurses to come to South Africa (Searle 1965: chs 7 and 9).

The Anglican sisters

The life of the settler group was *structured* around the family, which gave it stability. As the number of settlers increased and urban communities developed, health needs increased. The philosophy of health care in British Kaffraria, which advocated health services as a civilising influence, had far-reaching implications. Nor must the contribution of missionary work to health services be forgotten. The missionaries were of different denominations. A high standard of nursing was practised by the early British nurses. They were, according to the standards of the day, all educated women and laid a foundation upon which the Anglican Sisterhoods could build the formal training of nurses in South Africa.

In 1874 sisters of the first Anglican sisterhood to be established here arrived in South Africa. Sister Henrietta Stockdale, of the Sisterhood of St Michael and All Angels, started the formal training of general nurses in South Africa at the Carnarvon Hospital in Kimberley in 1877. This training formed the nucleus from which training schools as far afield as Barberton, Pretoria, Queenstown and Cape Town could draw trained personnel to establish their training programmes. By 1895 secular trainees from the school in Kimberley could take over the running of the hospital so that the religious sisters could withdraw. It is also to Henrietta Stockdale that we owe the fact that South Africa, in 1891, became the first country in the world to grant state registration to trained nurses.

By 1825 British people had settled in Natal and from their ranks came dedicated doctors and nurses who contributed their share to the development of nursing in South Africa. The settlers in Natal had their own specific health problems. They were confronted with cultural differences not only with the Zulu race, but also with the Indians, a new racial group with a new culture introduced into the country as indentured labour (Searle 1965: ch 10).

The training of Black nurses

It was also as a result of British settlement that the training of Black nurses was initiated. The beginnings were necessarily small, for the basic education of Black women was generally too limited to use as a foundation upon which to build professional education. Nevertheless, a start was made (Searle 1965: ch 9).

War with the Boer republics

The war between the English and the Boer republics waged at the turn of the century brought with it its share of misery, not least of which was the typhoid epidemic to which hundreds of troops fell victim. There was such gross lack of appreciation of the need for good camp hygiene that it was inevitable that health hazards which contributed to epidemics and many deaths. What trained nurses there were could not cope with the load of work, the totally inadequate facilities and the lack of food, water and equipment.

Some trained nurses did not measure up to standard, but most were devoted in their care of the sick and had to bear a burden that was very heavy indeed. Doctors were in even shorter supply than trained nurses and the latter often had to work without full-time medical officers. In these instances the trained nurse often assumed control of camp matters which were not military in nature, including schools.

The high death rate in the camps eventually prompted Lord Milner, spurred on by Emily Hobhouse and the Ladies' Commission, to ask for experienced matrons from England capable of training nurses and organising hospitals.

After the end of the South African War and the signing of the Treaty of Vereeniging, the two former Republics became British possessions and health legislation followed the same pattern as that already in existence in the Cape Colony and in the Colony of Natal. Thus British influence in nursing was widespread (Searle 1965: ch 14).

The legacy of 'gentle women' and payment

The British idea that 'gentle women' could not be employed for gain but could render service to the less fortunate led to the development of lady nurses who were motivated by the service element inherent in the work. It also meant that those who came forward for training were well-educated for their day. It also gave rise to inadequate remuneration, 'ladies' not being expected to need payment for their services. This latter idea was a long time in being eliminated from the minds of not only those responsible for paying nurses, but also nurses themselves, self-sacrifice, a vocational calling to service and little or no pay being part of the 'image' of the nurse that became firmly established in the minds of all concerned. The Victorian way of life in South Africa affected attitudes to the education of women and it was felt that families would 'support' girls. This had implications for the education of nurses in the twentieth century.

Miss BG Alexander of the Johannesburg Hospital was an enlightened British nurse who made a great contribution to nursing education in this country.

It was she who realised that the training of nurses should be based on community and national needs and not on the labour force needed to staff a particular hospital.

There is no doubt that the British made a significant contribution to the development of nursing and nursing education in South Africa. Today their descendants and those they trained form part of the South African nation, proud of its heritage which is a mixture of those of the nations that make up the conglomerate that exists today (Searle 1965: ch 19).

The Afrikaner nation

Formation

While all this was happening another phenomenon that was to shape the destiny of the land was occurring. The Afrikaner nation was slowly forming and gaining an identity and a language of its own.

The present Afrikaner folk of South Africa has a mixed ancestry. Simon van der Stel established 23 Dutch and German families in the Berg River Valley at Drakenstein. The French Huguenots who arrived in 1687 were settled at Drakenstein and Franschhoek, but they were interspersed with the other nationalities and were not allowed to form groups to preserve their French identity.

Amalgamation of these races took place. No further French settlers were admitted and the European elements were welded into a single people. French as a language in common use died out, but not before it had played its part in breaking down the spoken High Dutch of the late seventeenth century into the very earliest form of Afrikaans, which in 1925 was to receive formal recognition as an official language of the Union of South Africa. The Afrikaner nation, formed from Dutch stock with German, Belgian, French and later also British additions, came into being (Walker 1968: various sections).

Influence of religion

The people who came out to settle and the women who were sent out to marry them were Protestants. The early settlers had been involved in religious wars and were against oppression. They were very self-reliant. Their common bonds led to a closely knit community with marked group feeling and mutual helpfulness to members of their own group. They brought with them the influence of the narrow ethical codes of Calvinism and a presbytery system of church organisation.

The Church accepted responsibility for welfare services among the poor. Men in the community were expected to give attention to the spiritual welfare of people while women were expected to look after the sick. The deaconess system was followed and those performing social services and nursing were regarded as servants of the Church.

The Afrikaner nation was formed from a group of nations which regarded the midwife as being an important person in the social sphere. The midwife was seen as having many duties, including marriage guidance, advice to young people regarding marriage and its responsibilities, and health education. They were expected to determine whether a woman was pregnant, to ascertain her general state of health and to keep her in that state. They gave physical and emotional support during childbirth and their aim was a healthy mother.

Language problems

Language problems began to be experienced, especially when English became the official language. The movement that led to the Great Trek was under way. The Afrikaner nation was becoming welded together by the happenings of the times. The discovery of diamonds and the rush of foreigners or 'uitlanders' to the diamond fields brought about new health needs which were experienced yet again when gold was discovered. Hospitals were established to meet the health needs of these 'foreigners' and the Afrikaners were excluded. They looked after their own sick and were opposed to the idea of their daughters working for people of other nations.

The South African War

The South African War strengthened the feeling against foreign nurses. Afrikaner women coming out of the concentration camps were in a state of ill-health as a result of the despicable camp conditions, and this was aggravated by the extreme poverty to which they returned. The death and marriage registers of the time show a large number of female deaths and remarriage among widowers. The women's poor state of health contributed to the high death rate in childbirth, and because some of the blame was laid at the door of the 'ou tantes' doctors began to want trained nurses. The only ones available were British nurses who had remained behind. The Afrikaners could not accept them. Language difficulties and antagonism as a result of the War and the camps all contributed to this state of affairs and although the King Edward VII Order of Nurses instituted a form of district nursing service, this was not used by the people.

Afrikaner involvement in training

In 1918 the Helpmekaar Association started a movement which aimed at having a trained midwife in every community. Money was collected and selected girls were sent for training. Bodies such as the Suid-Afrikaanse Vrouefederasie, the Afrikaanse Christelike Vrouevereniging, the Natalse Christelike Vrouevereniging and the Oranje Vrouevereniging all played a part in sponsoring district nursing services. At first only qualified bilingual midwives were available, but they did general nursing as well and also undertook health education and social work.

To meet the need for Afrikaans speaking midwives the Suid-Afrikaanse Vrouefederasie established a maternity hospital, the Bond van Afrikaanse

Moeders Hospital, in Pretoria in 1918. It was sold to the Transvaal Provincial Administration in 1959. By that time bilingualism of nurses was an established fact. Nevertheless the pioneering work done by these Afrikaner women in providing for the needs of their people was of great importance, for they conditioned the Afrikaner to the need for skilled nursing and gave the nurse an honoured place in the community. The South Africa Act of 1909 provided equal language rights for English and Dutch speakers (Afrikaans as such was recognised as an official language in 1925).

First Afrikaner to train as a nurse

In 1886 an Afrikaner woman, Alice Eveline de Beer, came forward for training as a nurse in Kimberley. Sister Henrietta showed a great deal of interest in her progress, spending her own time teaching this young woman, for she hoped that other Afrikaner women would be persuaded to enter nurse training in order to meet the nursing needs of their own people.

Training through the medium of Afrikaans

Despite the language provisions of the South Africa Act, Afrikaans as a medium of instruction in nurse training was slow to get off the ground. The pioneer in this field was Miss Elizabeth Lotz of the National Hospital, Bloemfontein, who coached students in Afrikaans and compiled notes in that language which she made available to those she coached. In 1920 Miss Anna Schoeman took over this coaching in Afrikaans, although formal lectures were still in English.

In 1925 the Orange Free State Medical Council allowed two nurses to write the final examination for medical and surgical nurses in Afrikaans and to use that language for the oral and practical portion of the examination.

Afrikaans was introduced as a medium of instruction at the Somerset Hospital by Miss C Loopuyt. Later Miss Schoeman introduced it at the Far East Rand Hospital, Miss Alida Beyers at Pretoria, Miss W le Roux at Boksburg and Mrs C Searle at Klerksdorp. Pretoria University established a course for the training of nurse educators through the medium of Afrikaans and the use of Afrikaans as a medium of instruction spread rapidly throughout the country.

The early development of nursing education among Afrikaner girls was also limited by the lack of schools, teachers and suitable subject combinations. Nevertheless, great strides have been made and the Afrikaner nation has already produced leaders of quality from its ranks. As bilingualism has now become a way of life for South Africans and more and more blurring of race boundaries occurs, the future leaders, writers and teachers will come from a South African rather than a British or an Afrikaner background. They will produce the quality of nurse that the country as a whole needs, built on the best of both Afrikaner and British groups with a leaven from other races that have produced their common heritage.

The Black nations

The population of South Africa is of a multinational nature. There is no such thing as a single Black nation in the Republic. The term Black is generally applied to the dark negroid people who inhabit the southern part of Africa. They are distinguished from other population groups in Africa such as the Negroes, Hamites, Nilotes, Semites, Bushmen, Hottentots and Whites on both linguistic and cultural grounds.

Tongues used by the indigenous tribes include hundreds of languages and thousands of dialects. Because these possess a similarity in structure and syntax they are regarded as belonging to a language 'family'. The Black people do not form a homogeneous group, but consist of numerous separate peoples which can only be grouped together as forming a large 'family' according to very broad delineations. Some of the more important Black peoples of South Africa include the Xhosa, Zulu, Swazi, Sotho, Shangaan, Tsonga and Tswana, and they have different languages, dialects and cultures.

Contact with White settlers

The Black people did not come into contact with the White settlers of the Cape until late in the eighteenth century when White people began to venture into the interior. The Black people were cattle farmers who required extensive grazing lands for their herds. Thus they migrated southwards in search of more grazing. At the same time the trekboers were moving northwards with the same purpose as one of their reasons for leaving the original settlement. The Black peoples were more numerous and offered more resistance to White advance than had the Hottentots and Bushmen. The clash over grazing land that resulted between the frontier farmers and the Black races led to many years of frontier unrest and a series of frontier wars. (Broadly based on Walker 1968.)

Mission influence

At the same time missionaries had come out from England to the Cape Colony to work among the Hottentots and the Black tribes. These missionaries established isolated settlements in the interior. Their main objective was evangelical, but many of them realised that there was a need for care of the body that housed the soul should it become diseased. It was from these small beginnings that many mission hospitals originated.

In June 1820 the Rev John Brownlee established a mission station at Chumie near the present King William's Town. He paved the way for all the effective mission work in the Eastern Cape. Educational centres developed as a natural outcome of his work and these provided the nucleus of education for Black men and women that made possible the eventual education of Black nurses. Missionary efforts and mid-century 'Native' policy (Sir George Grey's idea of civilising the Blacks and the establishment of the Province of British Kaffraria between the Keiskamma and Kei rivers with its capital at King William's Town) all influenced the beginning of Black nursing. There was a regiment stationed at King William's Town which had attached to it highly experienced medical men. As there were no civilian doctors in the town during its early stages of development, the military medical personnel provided an emergency service for White civilians and for the Black peoples in times of need.

First hospital for Blacks

In 1856 the first hospital for the Black races was established on South African soil. Dr JP Fitzgerald was appointed Superintendent of Hospitals in British Kaffraria. He started his work in King William's Town by opening a clinic for the Black population. He had a tremendous task before him, for the Blacks tended to rely on their witch-doctors in times of illness and viewed 'White' medicine with suspicion. Many of these witch-doctors were skilled in the use of herbs and achieved success in the treatment of patients. It was many years before the Black people willingly entered hospitals. To this day they tend to consult witch-doctors as well as practitioners of 'White' medicine. No doubt they feel they are getting the best of both worlds.

The first Black people employed by the hospital as interpreters and hospital attendants were men. Dr Fitzgerald wanted assistants who could at least write and speak English. The male dominance in tribal life had led naturally to the Black males receiving what education was available.

The cattle killing

In 1857 came the great cattle killing when, according to a prophecy, it was promised that on an appointed day the Whites would be driven into the sea by a whirlwind, the dead heroes of the Black nation would arise from the earth followed by thousands of cattle, and corn would grow such as had never before been seen. The tribes were bidden to prepare for this miracle by sowing no corn and by killing and eating cattle. This they did, but no miracle occurred to save them and a starving people was left. Grey was prepared for this event with troops and food, but the resultant mortality among the starving hordes was dreadful. It is estimated that 50 000 Blacks died of starvation in the Ciskei alone.

Large stocks of food had also been laid down by Brownlee, but many of those affected by this disaster were too weak to reach the storage areas and died on the way. Soup kitchens and relief houses were organised by Dr Fitzgerald and Dr Willmans. A relief nursing service was provided by the ladies of King William's Town, and four Black women, who were the first to be employed as paid hospital nurses, were sent to assist at the hospital. The numbers soon increased (Searle 1965: ch 9).

Training of Black women

When the crisis period passed the point had been made that there was a place for Black women as nurses. Dr Fitzgerald obtained the services of Mrs Ellen Parsons, who was a widow with experience in nursing. In 1869 she was appointed to train Black women as nurses, a task she carried out for 22 years. The 'training' was elementary, including the rudiments of nursing, hygiene, nutrition and cooking for invalids. She taught them to read and write and to do arithmetic. From 1872 they also received instruction in the care of the lying-in woman (Searle 1965: 131).

Training Black women as nurses according to the 'Nightingale pattern' which had been established in other parts of the colony was not possible because of the lack of basic education among Black women. Although the credit goes to Lovedale Hospital for the preparation of the first Black auxiliary nurses, who were awarded hospital certificates, and the first Black professional nurse, Cecilia Makiwane, who was registered in 1908, it is to Dr Fitzgerald and Mrs Parsons that credit must go for the pioneering work they did in the field of nurse training for Black women. The nurses' register of the Colonial Medical Council was open to all race groups provided they could attain the desired standards in the examinations after undergoing an approved course of training. McCord Zulu Hospital in Durban commenced a course of nurse training similar to that run at Lovedale, that is a course that led to hospital certification. Training for Black professional nurses was commenced there in 1924, when suitable candidates first became available.

The training of Black professional nurses in sufficiently large numbers to meet the needs of their people and to make a significant contribution to nursing in South Africa as a whole did not really gain impetus until after the Second World War.

Black women with the educational background and mental outlook necessary for professional training were not available earlier for a variety of reasons, the most important of which were the following:

☐ Tribal prejudice
☐ Too short a period of contact with Western civilisation to have influence on their thinking
☐ Lack of sufficient secondary schooling facilities
☐ The male dominance in Black culture, which led to boys getting preference when secondary education facilities were available
☐ The drive by the Cape education authorities to absorb what Black women there were with secondary education into teacher training schemes
☐ The early marriage pattern of black women, and also the lobola system
☐ The use of Black hospital patients in urban areas for the training of White nurses
☐ Lack of uniformity and standards for the training of Black nurses
☐ Lack of definite policy with regard to the education of Black women as professional nurses (Searle 1965: chs 9, 15 and 17).

Auxiliary categories

The training of an auxiliary category of Black nurses had been proceeding in a rather haphazard fashion and in 1948 the provincial administrations of the Cape, Transvaal and Natal assumed responsibility for subsidising Black hospitals where courses of nurse training were given. Thus they took over subsidising Black nurse training from the South African Native Trust which, because there was such a need for Black nurses, subsidised any course, irrespective of its quality.

The provincial administrations, when they assumed control, began prescribing curricula and training conditions, inspecting training schools, conducting examinations and issuing provincial certificates of competency to Non-White auxiliary nurses. These certificates were given statutory recognition in 1957 when the Nursing Act made provision for the enrolment of auxiliary nurses of all race groups. In subsequent legislation this category became known as enrolled nurses, the 'auxiliary' title being dropped. Midwifery training for Black women commenced at McCord Zulu Hospital in 1927 and by 1960 49,3% of all Black registered nurses had a dual registration. By 1977 this figure was 15 155. It is interesting to note that in 1927 there were two registered Black female general nurses, in 1957 there were 433, in 1967 there were 7 853 and in 1977 there were 16 290 at the end of the year. The number of Black registered nurses on 31 December 1986 was 26 969 showing a continuing increase.

These tremendous improvements in the numbers of registered general nurses are attributable to various factors:

☐ An increased acceptance by the Black of White man's medicine, which led to an increase in the demand for hospital beds for Blacks
☐ Improvements in secondary educational facilities for Blacks
☐ The growing shortage of White nurses to meet the increased demand for Black health services
☐ The migration of Blacks from rural to urban areas, with the subsequent increased need for health services
☐ The policy of separate development, which gave Black nurses the opportunity to take over responsibility for running their own services
☐ Increased professional opportunities for qualified, registered Black nurses.

The first Black assistant matron was appointed in 1958. Today there are Black matrons of all categories, while specialisation courses in the various nursing disciplines have produced tutors, paediatric nurse specialists, community nurses, intensive care nurse specialists, operating theatre nurse specialists, ophthalmic nurse specialists and others. There are Black chief nursing officers and university lecturers and psychiatric training is now a compulsory component of the comprehensive course.

Many Black women are now making use of the opportunities afforded by the University of South Africa courses to further their nursing education and to take nursing degrees. University education for Black nurses has been available at post-basic diploma level for a considerable time. Post-basic degrees are also available at the University of the North. Basic degree courses in nursing for Black women are now becoming available, there being one in South Africa and one in Ciskei to date. Two doctorates in nursing have already been conferred and in 1987 two Black professors of nursing were appointed (Searle 1965: ch 17).

The disease pattern among the Black nations

Because of the socio-economic status of many Blacks, as well as their cultural patterns, lack of education and ignorance of hygiene practices and preventive medicine, including nutrition, Blacks are susceptible to a variety of diseases related to poor hygiene and sanitary arrangements, poor nutrition and other social factors. These patterns also show changes, as many urbanised Blacks are beginning to show 'Western-type diseases'.

Shortage of health personnel

There is a serious shortage of medical practitioners serving Black people and the number of Black medical practitioners is negligible. There has been a swing from tribal to scientific medicine and the burden of providing the types of health services needed and wanted has fallen largely on nurses, who often have to render primary health care under long-distance control of the physician leader of the team. Here the doctor has to be on tap. There is also an extreme shortage of pharmacists, radiographers, physiotherapists, laboratory technicians and occupational therapists; here again nurses have had to fill the gaps as best they can. The nurse's function as a health educator is also vital in providing health care. There has been a phenomenal increase in the Black population over the past 70 years. Much of this can be attributed to improved health services for Blacks.

Standards of nursing care

Black women have shown that they have the ability to attain standards of nursing care comparable with any in the world. With proper educational training they achieve high standards in national examinations. The improvement in the training of Black nurses has provided large numbers of competent, qualified personnel and this has been a continuous process. It has received stimulus from the development of the national states, which has given Black professional nurses the opportunity to take over their own nursing services and made them increasingly aware of the need for continuing education to fit them more adequately for their roles.

The Black registered nurse has proved her ability to take part in the shaping of policy. She has learnt to frame her thoughts and take part in debates by participation in professional activities.

Since 1979 Black nurses have served as members of the South African Nursing Council and since 1982 on the Central Board of the South African Nursing Association, as have Coloured and Indian nurses. The enrolled categories of the Black nursing profession have also played a significant part in providing badly needed health services to their people who, otherwise, would have been denied such health care.

The contribution that the registered Black professional nurse has already made and will make on an ever-increasing scale in the years that lie ahead is all the more remarkable when one realises that only 50 years elapsed between the registration of the first Black nurse and the appointment of the first Black matron, and since Black professional nurse training did not really get going to any extent until after 1948, it can be seen what remarkable feats have been achieved by Black nurses in the last 40 years, a very short time in the history of nursing. Their contribution to the health services as a whole has been of inestimable value to the entire population of the country (Searle 1965: chs 9, 18).

The Coloured group

The Coloured community, a small population group, comprising at present 2 832 705 (1985 census) people, live mostly in the Western Cape Province, where they have their origins. The Cape Peninsula was the centre of the Cape Coloured community, which monopolised certain areas even before the provisions of the Group Areas Act, but other fairly large communities are to be found in Port Elizabeth, East London and Johannesburg.

General education

Coloured schooling has in many instances been of a high standard and for many years students have had access to universities. They now boast their own University of the Western Cape which, with regard to the health services, trains dentists, nurses at basic degree, post-basic diploma level and degree level, and pharmacists. A medical school is in the planning stage. Other important disciplines available are social work, education, sociology and psychology, as well as the natural and biological sciences and librarianship. Nursing education for Coloured students commenced with midwifery training at St Monica's Hospital Cape Town in 1917. A few Coloured women also trained as general nurses at the Lovedale Hospital and were admitted to the Register of the Colonial Medical Council.

Nursing education

In 1938 the Cape Hospital Board came to the decision that increasing numbers of Coloured nurses and midwives should be trained. When the New Somerset Hospital was converted into a hospital for Coloured patients in July 1939, a training school for Coloured nurses was established there. Today others, such as the Coronation Hospital in Johannesburg and the Tygerberg Hospital in Bellville (Coloured section), as well as Groote Schuur Hospital (Non-White section), also train Coloured nurses. The Nico Malan Nursing College and the Sarleh Dollie College at Tygerberg Hospital cater for the educational needs of nurses. The training of Coloured nurses to serve their own population groups has not developed as rapidly as that of the Black nations. There are several reasons for this, including the following:

☐ Coloured education has provided students of a good quality, but diverse employment opportunity for these school-leavers has limited the number of Coloured girls entering nurse training

☐ Lack of training facilities, which have only recently become adequate.

At the end of 1986 there were 5 737 registered Coloured nurses in the Republic of South Africa. When this is seen against the 1 002 registered Coloured female nurses in 1960, then it is obvious that progress has been made, although there is still room for improvement.

Nurse leaders have emerged among the Coloured practitioners of nursing. They have developed their skills in policy-making spheres and are ready to play a direct role in the shaping of the South African nursing profession of the future. Although their numbers are small, they have a vital role to play (Searle 1965: ch 17).

The Indians

Mention must be made of the smallest population group of all, the Indian community, numbering at present 821 361 persons (1985 census). For various reasons, some of which are cultural, Indian women have been very slow to come forward for nurse training. The situation is improving gradually, but there is a long way to go before the distance is made up. In 1986 there were 1 386 Indian nurses on the registers of the South African Nursing Council. Leaders have emerged, although they are still few in number. Future developments will be watched with interest. There is no doubt that the contribution made by Indians will increase.

* * * *

Religion, wars, exploration and colonisation, social change, scientific and technological developments and the constantly evolving role of the nurse have all played a part in the development of nursing in South Africa.

3 Nature and evolution of specific types of nursing

GENERAL NURSING

Although this category of nurses is by far the largest group of practising nurses today, little space will be devoted to it in this work, for the development or evolution of nursing throughout the world refers in the main to the general nurse. Specific categories of nurses have evolved as a result of historical trends to meet specific needs. Many of these specialist categories started off when general nurses found and developed special interests in response to specific needs. Some of these specialist categories will receive separate attention. The generalist is so well known that it may seem superfluous to devote time and space to a discussion of general nursing.

Changing pattern

The nurse is concerned with man from birth to death. Some of her functions are specialised and additions and changes which have and may continue to lead to specialisation are made all the time. Nursing, being a dynamic profession, has not stood still. It will never stand still while human need exists.

The general nurse of today is very different from the general nurse of bygone days. Even Florence Nightingale would not recognise her, although she would acknowledge the qualities that are still necessary to make a successful general nurse. Perhaps now is the appropriate time to attempt to define what is meant by a general nurse – which is no easy task.

The professional general nurse is to be found in all communities, in all hospital wards, in clinics, in private homes and in doctors' consulting rooms. She is a professional nurse who has undergone a long period of basic training, passed the required examinations and been admitted to the register of her national body. She is competent to carry out nursing care of patients suffering from medical and surgical conditions except that which is of a highly specialised nature.

The general nurse is competent to observe and report on a patient's condition and obtain expert help when necessary. She is capable of applying primary health care in all normal circumstances and of recognising the need for care that is beyond her capabilities and ensuring that this is obtained as speedily as possible. She is capable of considered judgment and decision making in the nursing care context. She can make and implement nursing care plans. She can run a nursing care unit, teach personnel and patients, and more highly specialised, expert knowledge. The general nurse is prepared more highly specialised, expert knowledge. The general nurse is prepared at degree and diploma level. The comprehensive course no longer prepares a singly qualified general nurse, although at the end of 1986 there were still 11 381 general nurses with no further qualifications on the registers of the SANC. This number will decrease in time.

Advanced general nurse training

Just as the medical profession has recognised the need for special additional training for general practice, it has been recognised that the general nurse must receive more advanced training and recognition of her 'generalist' role. Many nurses leave ward work not because they want to do so, but because promotion opportunities lie elsewhere and promotion is important for financial reasons when pensionable service is considered.

More use should be made of an advanced general nursing certification. Financial recognition is also necessary if good general nurses are to be kept where they are happiest and of most use, that is with their patients in the clinical nursing field. The evolving role of the nurse applies to the general nurse as much as to the specialist nurse. The history, trends and evolution of the general nurse are basically the historical trends and evolution of nursing throughout the ages and stretch into the future.

Support from enrolled categories

The professional general nurse is helped and supported by other categories of nurses also working in the field of general nursing. In the South African situation these categories are the enrolled nurses and enrolled nursing assistants working in the fields of medical and surgical or general nursing. Their training is geared to complementing and aiding the work of the professional general nurse at a lower level. The enrolled categories of nurses are also found in specialist units where the specialist nurse with additional training takes the lead in nursing care.

MIDWIFERY

The art or practice of assisting women in childbirth must be one of the oldest forms of specialised help. As a vocation it has existed since time immemorial and has been practised almost exclusively by women.

Childbirth is a natural process and in the more primitive societies was and still is accompanied by as little interruption of the household duties of the mother as possible.

Early history

The care of the mother and baby has undergone extensive changes through the ages. Although childbirth and all that goes with it was a natural part of the life of primitive women, it was clothed in mystery and there were a multiplicity of gods and goddesses thought to be concerned with fertility and childbirth.

The Hebrews

Midwives are mentioned in the Bible. The Mosaic code prescribed strict measures regarding the hygiene of pregnancy, while Ezekiel described Hebrew birth practices.

The Hippocratic period

In the Hippocratic period, 470-370 BCE, Aphrodite and Artemis were regarded as goddesses concerned with fertility. The role of the priest-physician was later separated from that of the midwife and midwifery practice became well established during the Hippocratic era.

Unfortunately, the role played by the physician in the care of women in labour was not very great because it was not founded on any knowledge beyond that acquired in practice.

Greece and Rome

The type of care given to women in childbirth in Greece and later in Rome, where Greek medical influence was strong, developed considerably from that of primitive times and reached a peak in the writings of Soranus of Ephesus, who lived in the second century AD. His writings on obstetrics set standards of midwifery upon which no advance was made for 1 500 years. Later writers adapted his works.

Ireland

Another country which has left a record of midwifery practice is Ireland, which had a high degree of civilisation as early as 1 000 BCE and was one of the earliest countries to be converted to Christianity. Early practices in midwifery and obstetrics are recorded. The birth process was considered to be a normal event and was not attended by a physician, but the mother was assisted by a 'wise woman' or by her own mother. The Irish mother, like those of most other primitive cultures, was out of bed and back at her normal tasks within a short space of time.

Later developments

Midwifery and such obstetric practice as there was remained in the hands of midwives until early in the eighteenth century, although the names of William Harvey (1578-1657), the English physician who discovered the circulation of the blood, is known to have practised obstetrics and wrote on the subject in 1651, and the Chamberlens, a family of Huguenot refugees, figured in obstetrical history before that time. William Smellie (1697-1763) is often regarded as the father of British midwifery. He was born at Lanark in Scotland and studied medicine at Glasgow. Two years after settling in London he began to teach midwifery at his house.

Female midwives

In the seventeenth century the female midwife held a recognised social position and was sometimes not only well educated, but well paid. Midwifery 'training' in Britain was of an apprentice type and successful midwives were considered to be very little, if at all, inferior to the doctors of the time. The midwives had to be licensed.

Medical men's involvement

With the development of 'midwifery or obstetric practice' among doctors, the more affluent classes began to employ doctors in place of midwives. Queens were now attended by physicians instead of women skilled in the art of midwifery. Because of this lack of opportunity for midwives to carry out their former practice among the wealthy, the vocation of midwifery lost its well-paid, socially well placed members and thus also lost prestige. The work of attending the poorer members of society and assisting the obstetrician, who seldom saw his patient before labour began, was left to poorly educated women with little training of the Gamp type.

Victorian prudery also added to the lack of knowledge of midwifery, as the subject was considered 'indelicate' and therefore could not be aired in public.

Reform in midwifery

It was not until a few determined women, led by a Miss Louisa Hubbard, got together and founded the Midwives Institute in 1881 that matters began to improve.

Central Midwifery Board in Great Britain

In 1902 the Midwives Act, which protected the title of midwife and limited the practice of midwifery so that the profession became virtually closed, was passed. The Act set up a Central Midwives Board to keep a register of midwives, to make rules for the conduct of midwifery and to set minimum standards of professional education and behaviour. This laid the foundation for the present practice of midwifery in Britain by trained, registered and supervised women. British midwives today are independent practitioners.

During this period medical developments which affected midwifery practice were the introduction of the use of anaesthesia in midwifery by the obstetrician James Young Simpson in 1847 and the theory of the cause of puerperal fever put forward by Ignaz Philipp Semelweiss (1818-1865) in Vienna (others who worked in this field were Alexander Gordon and Oliver Wendell Holmes). It remained for Pasteur in 1879, 14 years after the death of Semelweiss, to prove what before had been only supposition based on clinical observation. Thus maternal mortality due to puerperal sepsis began to be controlled as aseptic practices were introduced into midwifery. The cure for puerperal sepsis was found in 1930 with the discovery of antibiotics.

Preventive medicine

Later developments in the practice of midwifery were the establishment of preventive medicine as part of midwifery practice. Antenatal supervision became normal practice. With the establishment of the Royal College of Obstetricians and Gynaecologists, obstetrics became a branch of medicine in its own right. Obstetrics was a compulsory subject in the training of doctors. The discovery of the rhesus factor in the blood and the effects of incompatibility on the child has, with further research and modern treatment, almost eliminated erythroblastosis foetalis.

Ante-partum and post-partum haemorrhage can be prevented or dealt with by modern methods of monitoring patients and blood transfusion. Toxaemia of pregnancy can be recognised early and controlled. Babies can be monitored before birth so that early signs of foetal distress can be noted and dealt with by Caesarean section or other methods before the baby is damaged. Vacuum extractions are possible. Ultrasound and cardiotocography are practised, as are diagnostic tests such as amniocentesis. Midwifery practice changes with increased medical knowledge and will continue to do so.

South African perspectives

The trends in midwifery practice in South Africa will now be highlighted in order to place them in perspective.

Historical overview

Indigenous people

We must now turn our attention to the state of affairs prevailing in this country in so far as the history of midwifery can be traced.

With regard to the indigenous population of this country the roles of the witchdoctor and the traditional birth attendant are still enough in evidence to be understood by all of us. Some practices were primitive to say the least, if not positively dangerous. The treatment of the cord, the placenta, the puerperium and lactation varied according to the place and the tribe. Maternal and child mortality occurred, but it must be remembered that these also occurred with alarming frequency among the so-called more civilised Western nations. There was a general lack of knowledge regarding childbirth, a situation which changed only with the upsurge of scientific inquiry in both the medical and nursing fields.

White settlement

With the founding of the White settlement in South Africa in 1652 we have some record of birth practices. The Hottentot woman who gave birth, unattended, close to the fort on the banks of the river on 18 April 1654, is described in Van Riebeeck's diary (Searle 1965: 28). This caused so much surprise that it can safely be assumed that Dutch women were used to receiving help and care from others when delivering their children and during the lying-in period.

Dutch East India Company regulations

It is recorded history that it was the policy of the Dutch East India Company to appoint official midwives to the trading stations in the East. There were specific regulations to control such midwives and these were applied at the Cape as soon as Jan van Riebeeck landed there. Embodied in them were the requirements that midwives should be in possession of certificates granted by examination. Midwives then, as now, had to be licenced to practise.

Midwifery services were regarded as a fundamental component of health care. Provision was made for competent assistance during childbirth for those who could not afford to pay. In the beginning midwifery practice was a service rendered in the homes of the settlers and in the slave lodge in Cape Town. It was, in effect, either a type of 'private practitioner' or State District service. The policy of the Dutch East India Company was to provide sworn midwives who usually came from the Netherlands to practise at the Cape. Some local women were also licensed from time to time.

British occupation

The administration and organisation of the Cape was considerably disorganised by the First British Occupation which lasted from 1795 to 1803. When control of the Cape returned to Dutch hands (1803-1806), the Batavian Republic authorities realised that there was a serious shortage of sworn midwives and planned to establish a midwifery training school there. However, there was again a change of control, the British re-occupying the Cape in 1807. This time the British began to pay attention to the health services and set up a Supreme Medical Committee charged with the examination of the qualifications and licencing of doctors and apothecaries. This was later extended to include midwives. Jean Martin, a male ex-surgeon, was refused a licence to practise as a surgeon and was licensed to practise as an 'accoucheur' only.

Training

Early efforts – Dr Wehr

The training of midwives on a systematic basis in the Cape actually owes its origins to Dr Johann Heinrich Frederick Carel Leopold Wehr, a surgeon of the Batavian authorities who became licenced to practise as a physician, surgeon and an accoucheur in 1805. He was extremely interested in midwifery and became very anxious about the type of midwifery practised by unlicenced persons. He thought it to be not only inadequate, but highly dangerous. In 1808 he wrote a petition to the British Governor-General and Commander-in-Chief of the Cape, pointing out that there was a great lack of 'proper and able midwives' in the Colony. He also stated the consequences to the health of mothers and children that resulted from this. He asked for appointment as colonial accoucheur and with it permission to instruct 'an adequate number of midwives for the town of each district'.

This office would also enable him to assist, without charge, the wives and slaves of poor inhabitants. Permission was granted on 1 August 1808.

The Supreme Medical Committee, in consultation with Dr Wehr, drew up regulations for the training of midwives and the establishment of a midwifery training school. Dr Wehr was appointed colonial instructor of midwifery on 1 November 1810 and shortly afterwards preparations were made to commence with such training.

South African midwifery training forerunner

This first midwifery school in South Africa was established on a formal basis 51 years before the St Johns Hospital midwifery school at Kings College in 1861 (Searle 1965: 95). The first midwives to complete a full-time course of training did so by 2 August 1813. These women were the first to qualify as professional people in any field of nursing in South Africa and the school was also the first professional school of any kind in South Africa. Students were taken from country districts as well as from Cape Town. Non-Whites were trained together with Whites for the service of their own people.

Hospital beds for midwifery

The first hospitals had no beds for midwifery cases. The first official mention of such beds being made available seems to have been at the Albany Hospital in Grahamstown in 1858 (Searle 1965: 102). Gradually it became the practice to provide beds in general hospitals for midwifery of an emergency nature.

The next phase – state registration

Sister Henrietta Stockdale, the pioneer of nursing registration in this country and, incidentally, in the world, was instrumental in obtaining registration for midwives at the same time as this was obtained for nurses. The passage of the *Medical and Pharmacy Act*, 1891 (Act 34 of 1891) by the Parliament of the Cape Colony made provision, *inter alia*, for the registration of midwives.

Regulations for training were promulgated on 31 May 1892. The first persons to register as midwives did so on the grounds of overseas qualifications. The regulations made provision for training under the direction of a medical practitioner. This made the formal reintroduction of midwifery training possible.

Mary Hirst Watkins is generally recognised as the founder of modern midwifery training in South Africa. In 1892 she was one of the first registered nurses in the world, having trained at the Kimberley Hospital. She continued to work at this hospital and in 1892 was assigned to midwifery district work by Sister Henrietta. Mary Hirst Watkins was trained in midwifery by local doctors and under the supervision of Sister Henrietta and Sister Catherine

Booth. The latter was trained in London as a general nurse and midwife and registered in South Africa on 6 September 1892.

Mary Hirst Watkins passed the midwifery examination of the Colonial Medical Council (in Port Elizabeth) in 1893 and was admitted to the register. She was then asked by Sister Henrietta to undertake the training of midwives at Kimberley. This she did, establishing a school which became famous.

Other midwifery training was also instituted. Dr Jane Waterson started a district midwifery service at the Free Dispensary in Cape Town in 1888 and trained midwives herself, but none of them sat the examination of the Colonial Medical Council and therefore were not registered. Registration of midwives first occurred in the Transvaal in 1896 and in Natal in 1899.

The twentieth century

A good foundation had been laid for midwifery training, but much remained to be done. Childbirth was a normal part of everyday life and midwifery care was needed. The sparse population was distributed over wide areas and there were insufficient medical men to meet the obstetrical needs of the community. More and more trained midwives were (and today still are) needed.

Duration of course

This has fluctuated from six months to the present integrated, comprehensive approach, of which midwifery is a compulsory component.

Number of registered midwives

It is interesting to note that at the end of 1986 there were 51 774 registered midwives in the Republic of South Africa. This group comprised 22 338 Whites, 5 087 Coloureds, 1 169 Indians and 23 180 Blacks, and of this number 516 were registered only as midwives. This shows a remarkable growth from the 62 registered by the Colonial Medical Council in 1899.

Changes in emphasis in certain subject matter

Modern developments have made certain changes in emphasis necessary. These have occurred in the fields of family planning and mothercraft, which have, for a long time, formed part of midwifery training. Care of the infant is as vital as care of the mother. Promotive and preventive health care is equally important.

Stitching and episiotomies

It is a fact that in the past midwives have often been called upon to do episiotomies and to stitch perineums. It is now part of the curriculum.

The advent of the male midwife (accoucheur)

The South African Nursing Council's decision to allow males to undertake midwifery training raised protests, although there was also much commendation of the move. Males delivering babies is nothing new, and the intimate care sometimes required of the midwife can be delegated to others.

The training of male midwives is in its infancy in this country, although not in others, and like all new things must be allowed to stand the test of time.

Other countries

Now that we have examined the development of midwifery in general, with particular emphasis on British midwifery, and studied midwifery in the South African context, it is necessary to look briefly at midwifery practice in other parts of the world as part of the study of the ethos of nursing.

Types of persons practising midwifery

Countries that were colonised tended to follow the pattern of midwifery practised by the colonising power. Development in midwifery education, as in general nurse education, was limited by the education facilities available to the indigenous population of the areas in question. The type of persons who practise midwifery and the functions of those, apart from physicians, who attend women in labour, show many variations and include the following:

The fully trained midwife The technical competence of the fully trained midwife extends beyond that required of a person who is of assistance at the time of delivery. She is expected to have the knowledge and skill to give total care to the mother and baby during pregnancy, labour and the puerperium. She must be able to detect the abnormal and the potentially abnormal and know what action to take in these situations. She must be able to educate and supervise the pregnant woman in health matters relating to her pregnancy and to supervise the health of the child and, to some measure, of the rest of the family. She must be able to function as a member of a team or independently. The fully trained midwife, with few exceptions, is common to most countries of the world.

The traditional birth attendant She has many names, including *dai, dayah, dukun, matrone* and *curiosa*. She is part of the social pattern of the underdeveloped areas and is the forerunner of the trained midwife, who came about as a historical development of the traditional birth attendant. The traditional birth attendant has a good deal of experience in the occupation she has chosen, but is often illiterate and may be steeped in traditional practices that conflict with modern midwifery knowledge and practice, so that she can actually cause harm to the mother and child.

Auxiliary midwife This type of worker may or may not be literate, being a traditional birth attendant who has been given some training. Where the education of women has reached a more advanced level, but has not yet progressed sufficiently for full midwifery training to be undertaken, the auxiliary midwife can be given a measure of training in antenatal and post-natal care, as well as in the perinatal care of the mother and baby. Thus she fills a gap in the health services, enabling the thin layer of midwives to be spread wider so as to serve more people.

Patterns of midwifery practice

Midwifery practice involves a wide range of activities, from the very primitive to the most sophisticated. The pattern of midwifery services has

developed along different lines in different countries so that the following variations are to be found:
- [ ] Areas where 90% of confinements take place in a hospital where the woman in labour is attended either by a physician and an obstetrical nurse, a physician and a midwife, or a midwife with a physician on tap for emergencies
- [ ] Areas where the majority of normal confinements take place in the home with perhaps a doctor, but more frequently a midwife, in attendance
- [ ] Large underdeveloped areas where the only attendant is a relative or an untrained traditional birth attendant who earns a poor living by giving service at the time of delivery
- [ ] Grey areas which fall between the underdeveloped and the highly developed areas.

Variations in practice

Customs, cultural patterns and traditional beliefs cause many variations in practices relating to pregnancy, childbirth and the care and management of the newborn. Rural and urban areas also influence midwifery services. European midwifery practice was taken to the Americas by the Pilgrim Fathers in 1620. The wife of Samuel Fuller, a deacon of the church who also acted as a physician, was the colony's first midwife. Anne Hutchinson and Ann Eliot, the wives of prominent men, also practised midwifery.

Oliver Wendell Holmes, appointed professor of anatomy at Harvard Medical School in 1840, was one of the first to analyse and point out the defects in obstetrical care and to stress the need for cleanliness to prevent the spread of infection.

During the mid eighteenth century there were many 'monthly' (obstetric) nurses who left much to be desired as midwives. It is interesting to note that while the development of general nurse education has received so much attention the United States of America, that of midwifery has been neglected. New Mexico has a law requiring state registration for midwives, who must be registered nurses who have followed an approved course in midwifery.

The first organised midwifery service in the USA was started in Kentucky by Mary Breckenbridge in 1925. She had to make use of English trained nurse midwives because there were so few such persons in America. These midwives often travelled long distances on horseback to assist women in labour who lived in remote areas.

Although the training of midwives *per se* is gaining momentum, one million women in the United States deliver babies annually without the attendance of a physician, and a quarter of a million are attended by untrained women. It will take time to remedy this situation, but the call for the training of nurse midwives is coming from obstetricians, and this is adding impetus to such training programmes. (SA references broadly based on sections of Searle 1965: chs 4, 5, 6, 7, 12, 18 and 19.)

PSYCHIATRIC NURSING

This branch of nursing began to receive recognition only in the late nineteenth and early twentieth centuries. Psychiatry, as a discipline of medicine, was an equally late development. Today psychiatry deals with personal, social and ethical problems in life that have their origin in disturbed interpersonal relationships.

From the earliest times deviations from the accepted norms of behaviour and the occurrence of mental disorders have been associated with demoniac possession, with sin, evil and the wandering of the soul or vital spirit from the body. The insane were classed in law next to criminals and their treatment ranged from indifference and neglect to gross brutality. These atrocities were perpetuated until the mid nineteenth century.

Reform movements

During the eighteenth century concern about the treatment of the insane started to gain momentum, and in England an attempt to regulate private institutions for the care of the mentally disturbed was made in 1774. The Act proved very difficult to enforce and did little to correct existing abuses. It also did not apply to public hospitals or institutions for the mentally deranged.

Another occurrence in English history that affected attitudes towards the mentally disturbed was the illness of George III, who was afflicted by intermittent bouts of mental disturbance. It is now believed that his illness was porphyria, which today would be treatable, but the fact that the King was afflicted by a mental disorder brought about changes in public thinking.

Pioneers in the movement for reform of the care of the mentally disordered included Mlle le Gras, superior of the order of St Vincent de Paul, who organised the humane care of the mentally ill as early as 1645. However, this was an isolated instance. In 1791 William Tuke, a well-known Quaker, became interested in the plight of the insane and persuaded the Society of Quakers to found a hospital, known as a 'Retreat', where humane treatment for the insane would be instituted.

Lord Ashley devoted much time and effort to the care of the insane, the Lunacy Act of 1845 being largely the result of his efforts.

Phillippe Pinel (1745-1826) was a Frenchman to whom credit must go for the removal of chains from patients and the introduction of humane methods of treatment for the mentally disordered. His chief scientific work was the classification of mental diseases according to symptomology.

Dorothea Lynde Dix (1802-1887), an American pioneer crusader for the reform of the treatment of the mentally ill, was instrumental in bringing about many changes and reforms.

Clifford W Beers (1876-1943) became mentally ill as a young graduate and was confined for three years to various institutions for the care of patients suffering from mental illness. His treatment varied from indifference to actual cruelty and his experiences during this period made him determined, when he recovered and was discharged, to devote himself to improving the lot of the mentally ill. He was instrumental in founding a local society and later a national committee for mental hygiene.

Need for trained psychiatric nurses

As these changes were occurring in the care of the mentally ill, as well as in medical attitudes towards this type of illness, a group of nurses specialising in the nursing of psychiatrically disturbed patients became established. Together with better-prepared psychiatrists, trained clinical psychologists, psychiatric social workers and occupational therapists, great strides have been made, in a comparatively short time, in this field of medicine and nursing. Modern treatment methods, including the use of tranquillisers, antidepressive drugs, modification of environmental factors which have a bearing on mental disorders (including physical illness and stress factors), electroconvulsive therapy, psychoanalysis and psychotherapy, group therapy, occupational and industrial therapy, are employed to manage these patients so that many are now successfully treated, discharged and maintained in the community as useful members of society.

Today psychiatric nursing is considered, along with general nursing, community nursing and midwifery, to be one of the basic disciplines of nursing.

Psychiatric nursing in the South African context

Custodial care

The attitude to the mentally ill at the Cape Colony was not coloured by such inhuman practices as existed in Western Europe, although there were poor facilities for insane paupers. During the jurisdiction of the Dutch East India Company the mentally ill were not ill-treated, and only those who became violent were locked up. Relatives of the more affluent looked after their own, incarcerating them when necessary. Those who were not violent were allowed to wander at will. Dangerous pauper lunatics were locked up in the slave lodge, where conditions were far from ideal. Nevertheless they were not abused and were visited daily by a barber-surgeon. During the Batavian Republic this system continued.

After the British occupation in 1806 conditions deteriorated for a while, the seriously insane being admitted to gaols and housed with criminals. When appointed Inspector of Lepers, the 'Tronk' and the Somerset Hospital in 1824, Dr James Barry attempted to bring about reform and eventually built up a pattern of care of the insane with a small core of reasonably satisfactory attendants and keepers.

First lunatic asylum

The Somerset Hospital became the lunatic asylum of the Cape Colony. Treatment was essentially of a custodial nature. It was not until the establishment of an asylum for the mentally ill on Robben Island in 1846 that a proper mental nursing service could develop. The pattern of care was humane and conditions were clean and reasonably congenial.

A cottage attached to the Albany General Hospital in Grahamstown was established for the reception of mentally disturbed patients, the nurses attending to general patients also assuming responsibility for the mentally ill. This ideal situation came to an end when in 1872 the British pattern of strict segregation of the mentally and physically ill was adopted. However, many more facilities, including those for the care of feeble-minded children, were provided and humane care continued to be the order of the day. Superintendents of hospitals consistently reported favourably on the good work done by nursing staff; their activities included much to lighten the lot of those committed to their care. Some training appears to have been given to nursing personnel by superintendents and senior nurses. Dr Thomas Duncan Greenlees, who was Superintendent of the Grahamstown Lunatic Asylum, launched the training of mental nurses in South Africa. The first certificate to be granted in the Cape was awarded in 1895.

Registration

The registration of trained nurses which was achieved in 1891 made it possible for a trained and duly qualified mental nurse to be registered, and accordingly in 1901 regulations were made for the granting of certificates to and the registration of mental nurses. However, the education of mental nurses got off to a very slow start indeed. Mental nursing had not yet achieved the respectability that general nursing had gained among the British, and it was completely foreign to Afrikaner culture in those early days.

Training

Eventually courses were established for mental nurses and nurses for mental defectives. The calibre of student attracted was not high and mental nursing was by-passed by the more educated persons planning to make nursing a career. Regulations for the training of psychiatric nurses were promulgated in 1954, but it was many years before a course leading to this qualification was introduced. Today there was 6 725 female and 525 male psychiatric nurses of all race groups on the register of the South African Nursing Council, while there are some on the registers (which are now closed) of mental nurses and nurses for mental defectives.

Gradual improvements were made to the courses leading to registration as a mental nurse, including a common preliminary examination for general nurses. The educational entrance requirements have also been brought in line with those of other registrations.

Psychiatric nurses

The introduction of psychiatric nursing on an integrated basis into degree courses for nurses has given impetus to psychiatric nursing in this country.

51

A number of students educated in this way have remained in psychiatric nursing. There are now nurses who hold a master's degree in psychiatric nursing. Although the numbers are small, they represent a significant development in psychiatric nursing in this country.

The Mental Health Act

The *Mental Health Act*, 1973 (Act 18 of 1973), which was promulgated in March 1975, was a significant development in the care of the psychiatrically ill and replaced legislation that had not been altered fundamentally since 1916.

The specific role of the psychiatric nurse as a link between the patient, his family and other members of the therapeutic team is based on the philosophy as well as the specific provisions of the new Mental Health Act. This ensures that the interests of the mentally ill patient are always regarded as paramount and that the relatives of the patient are correctly informed of the protection afforded them and the patient by the Act. Psychiatric nursing in South Africa has come of age and is now a compulsory component of the comprehensive course. (SA references broadly based on sections of Searle 1965: chs 8 and 19.)

COMMUNITY NURSING

The art and science of nursing has developed in response to social needs. The history of man has shown a continuous though erratic pattern of change in society. As society changes, new health care needs arise. New habits and customs which alter the pattern of disease develop with the passage of time, and changes in the numbers and grouping of the population lead to new patterns of community living, for example the development of urban areas. These bring about new health problems, including those caused by overcrowding, an inadequate water supply and sanitation. Society has to meet new health needs, which may arise very slowly or very rapidly, if it is to survive. How it meets them will vary according to the stage of development of the state, the economic resources, knowledge and manpower available, and the effect of cultural patterns on the society involved.

Medicine and nursing are commonly referred to as very old professions, yet modern medicine and modern nursing can hardly be considered more than a century old. Indeed, what was considered good practice a decade ago is today often looked upon with scorn. Nevertheless it is true that man has been concerned with health and health matters for a very long time. This concern has taken different forms, but has been linked to social concern and social reforms, including public education, public welfare, the care of the young, the care of the mentally ill, the care of the aged and many other aspects that are linked to the community aspects of medicine and nursing.

Historical perspective

Through reading history it is interesting to discover that many ancient civilisations had laws that were, in effect, sound health practices. Little is known about the origins of either personal or community hygiene in the pre-Christian period, but they probably grew up as a result of group and community experience and practice which enabled them to survive. Many primitive tribes have customs such as burying excreta and elaborate provisions for disposing of the dead. An example is that of the Zoroastrians, who fastened the body of the dead person to the roof of a specially high tower, where the birds picked the bones. These practices were based on custom and superstition, but they were effective. The Minoans (3000-1500 BCE) and the Cretans (3000-1000 BCE) had constructed drainage systems, water closets and water-flushing systems. The Egyptians of about 1000 BCE also had earth closets and public drainage systems and Herodotus stated that they were the healthiest of all civilised nations. They built granaries for storing food and water storage was practised. Midwifery was an established vocation.

The Hebrews

The Hebrews were well versed in community health practices, and the statements in the Books of Moses that describe personal and community responsibilities have a distinct bearing on health.

The Greeks

The culture of the Greeks, especially that of the Athenians, developed a degree of hygienic usage not previously achieved. Cleanliness, exercise, diet and environmental sanitation all received a great deal of attention. One significant public health practice which is in marked contrast to the attitude of today is that the weak, the ill and the crippled were ignored, if not deliberately destroyed. Weak, crippled infants were exposed to expedite death.

The Romans

The Romans were also advanced in measures having bearing on the health of the community, including the inspection and elimination of dilapidated buildings, the removal of dangerous animals and noxious odours, the supply of good grain at a cheap price and public sanitary services, which were of a high order.

Christian era

Although the early Christian era brought a reaction against care of the body, and 'mortification of the flesh' was a practice that led to a lowering of standards of hygiene and of sanitation which in turn caused the great epidemics of the Middle Ages, it was nevertheless part of the Christian ethic that the sick and suffering should be cared for. The early Christians sold all they possessed and gave to the poor. The Church was the central organisation for dispensing charity and the church worker, who distributed food and medicines to the needy in the community, became established. She gave care to those in need (such as bathing the sick, dressing wounds), fed the hungry, gave fluids to the sick and offered spiritual support to the ill and the dying.

Phoebe, the first deaconess, was probably the first visiting nurse. St Elizabeth of Hungary is another figure from the past who had a connection with community care. The Beguines of Flanders gave care to the sick of the community in their homes.

The Middle Ages were indeed dark ages characterised by much human suffering. Plagues and epidemics were rampant and medical knowledge appears to have been almost non-existent. The need for social reform was also great. St Francis de Sales and Madame de Chantal founded the Order of the Visitation of Mary in 1610. Madame de Chantal was its first superior. This order consisted of influential women who visited the sick in their homes, cared for their physical needs and dressed their wounds. They gave clothes to the needy sick and took their linen home for cleansing. This order was thus also one which worked in the community.

The next pioneer in this field was Vincent de Paul, who lived in France from 1581 to 1660. He was responsible for founding various bodies, but the one that affected nursing most was the 'Dames de Charité'. It was devoted to the care of the sick in their own homes.

Mlle Louise le Gras, later Madame de Marillac, became the first supervisor of these visiting nurses, accompanying them on their rounds. These women were mostly married women of high social standing. Eventually Les Filles de Charité (the daughters of charity), a non-cloistered religious order, was established. The women of this order wore the peasant dress of the day, which became symbolic of their order. They were young and full of enthusiasm and were trained by Louise de Marillac for this work, which grew and spread throughout the civilised world.

From the foregoing it will be seen that throughout nursing history people have been cared for in the community, that is in their own homes. This is also evident in the care of women in childbirth, which has been outlined in the section on midwifery. Social conditions in the cities of Europe during the eighteenth and early nineteenth centuries were deplorable. Hundreds of thousands of people lived in habitations that were appalling from a hygienic standpoint, so that diseases such as smallpox, cholera, typhoid, typhus, tuberculosis and many others took a dreadful toll on health and life. The loss of life, of work hours, and production due to disease was extremely high.

Legislation

It was as late as 1837 in England that the first legislation having a bearing on sanitary reform was passed. This was followed in 1848 by the establishment of a general board of health for England. Advances also began to be made in Europe, notably in the Low Countries, France, Germany and Scandanavia. British influence was felt in Colonial America. Thus public health services which over the decades had an ever-increasing influence on the health of the community, were established.

In the pattern that she established as the foundation of modern nursing, Florence Nightingale not only trained nurses for hospitals or to train others, but also to do district nursing among the sick poor. Gradually a division grew up in nursing, so that there was hospital nursing, private duty nursing and district nursing.

In England William Rathbone, whose wife died in 1859 despite every care, became aware of the plight of poor families who had no money and no help in times of illness. He was convinced of the need for a nursing service in the community and, with the help of Mrs Mary Robinson, established a nursing service in the community.

Eventually special training for district nurses was instituted, largely thanks to the efforts of Miss Lees, who had been a pupil of Florence Nightingale, and in 1889 The Queen Victoria Jubilee Institute for Nurses ('Queen's Nurses') was founded, providing special training for district work and for those who would work in rural areas.

School nursing

School nursing, a branch of community nursing, was introduced into the school system of London in 1892.

Tuberculosis nursing

Tuberculosis nursing, to meet the special needs of the time, also developed at the beginning of the twentieth century.

Industrial nursing

Industrial nursing was another type of community care that developed as the health of the workers came to be of concern to employees and the public.

From these beginnings grew the need for more and more specially educated nurses to meet community needs, the emphasis being on preventive work by all categories of health care workers. There is a shortage of health care manpower of all types throughout the world, and the categories of workers brought into the health team in many parts of the world are many and varied. They depend on the needs of the countries and the developmental and educational level of their peoples. There is a tremendous awareness of health needs throughout the world and governments are making great efforts to meet these needs. Training in community health care has been increasing significantly throughout the world, both in quantity and scope. Many former scourges have been brought under control. Maternal and child care has reduced both maternal and infant mortality.

The work of the World Health Organisation (WHO) has helped the countries which have very serious health problems and economic difficulties to launch and carry out programmes, all of which have contributed significantly to improvements in health. Large numbers of people who would previously have been incapacitated and thus unproductive, as well as a burden on state finance, have been kept well, active and productive. This means that the economies of countries have been improved by increased production instead of being weakened by a large number of persons in the population too ill or weak to work to their full potential. In all this preventive work the nurse, as a member of the health team, has played a vital role.

The future of health care everywhere depends on the prevention of preventable diseases. The fact that a mere 10% of diseases treated today are treated in hospital and that 90% are managed in the community is also an indication of the importance of the health worker in the community. The role of the community nurse is evolving in the same way as that of the nurse engaged in the curative field. Community nursing is just as vital and specialised a branch as any other form of nursing that has developed in response to health care needs.

Modern community nursing

The modern concept of community nursing has grown out of the past. The modern community nurse is seen as a well-prepared professional nurse with many facets to her practice, capable of giving comprehensive care. She is to be found in many fields of nursing, including district nursing, occupational health nursing, health visiting, psychiatric community nursing, school nursing, orthopaedic nursing, paediatric nursing, midwifery and others. She is the true practitioner of comprehensive nursing care, moving out from the purely curative orientation to the preventive, promotive and rehabilitative areas of health care. Community nursing is all-embracing. It is concerned with the total health care of the community, although it may be practised in different forms.

The therapeutically orientated hospital nurse also plays a part in comprehensive community care. Her patient comes from the community and hopefully will return to his usual environment, often after a very short stay in hospital. His episode of illness may even have its origins in the community. Community nursing is often considered to be the only type of nursing involved in preventive and promotive health care, yet this is a fallacy, for it is to be found in all fields. The nurse who is engaged in treating a 'patient' in hospital aims at:

☐ *preventing* complications
☐ *preventing* regression
☐ *promoting* recovery.

Rehabilitation also plays a part.

In many instances it is not possible to cure someone completely, but his condition can be arrested, his acceptance of limitations *promoted*, further deterioration *prevented* and he can be rehabilitated into the community. Health education is given to patients, their families and those who are concerned with their care.

Even when entirely hospital based, the midwife is very much involved in preventive and promotive health care, being engaged in preventing damage to the mother and child throughout pregnancy, labour, the puerperium and afterwards and of promoting the health of both. Health education is an important aspect of her function.

Many misconceptions about community nursing exist and many people believe that community nursing is practised only by those who are called public health nurses or health visitors, that is nurses employed by local authorities for a specific purpose. This concept has been restrictive and it is hoped that, with the general broadening of the concept of medicine as a comprehensive discipline and the ever-increasing interest in social medicine as such, the community nurse will be seen as 'any nurse concerned with rendering the nursing component of health care so that all members of the community can be afforded the opportunity to enjoy complete physical, mental and social well-being, and not only be free from disease or deformity'. If this broad view of what community nursing entails is taken, then it will be seen that nursing in the community is very old indeed.

Community nursing in the South African context

The view of what constitutes community nursing in this country has for a long time been as restricted as in many other lands. The term 'public health nurse' has come to mean those nurses employed by local authorities, particularly those with an additional qualification as a 'health visitor'. This erroneous demarcation has made the important roles played by the district nurse and midwife, the school nurse, the occupational health nurse, the nurse giving domiciliary geriatric care, in fact any nurse who has any connection with people in their community setting, go unappreciated.

The move by the South African Nursing Council to incorporate various aspects of nurse training into the post-registration diploma leading to registration as a community nurse and the incorporation of the discipline of community nursing into university nursing courses are commendable changes in thinking which should do much to rectify erroneous conceptions. The comprehensive diploma course now includes community nursing in the basic course for registration. The university degree courses which prepare students for registration are also comprehensive.

There are various milestones in the development of the community nursing service in this country which include the following:

☐ *The work of the four 'vroueverenigings'* The work of the 'Suid-Afrikaanse Vrouefederasie', the 'Afrikaanse Christelike Vrouevereniging (ACVV)' in the Cape, the 'Natalse Christelike Vrouevereniging' in Natal, and the 'Oranje Vrouevereniging' in the Orange Free State among the Afrikaner people as early as 1902 led to the establishment of district nursing and midwifery services, particularly in rural areas. The debt that community health care owes to these organisations is inestimable.

☐ *The district nursing service* This was established in 1912 by the Cape Hospital Board. The aim of this service was to improve the health of the community by providing health education, primary health care in homes or at clinics and a domiciliary midwifery service.

☐ *The contribution of voluntary organisations* Besides the 'vroueverenigings', there are other voluntary organisations that have made an indelible mark on the history of community health services in the country. They were established mainly to render social service, but as health could not be separated from social conditions they developed health services as part of their social service motive. Among the voluntary organisations was the King Edward VII Order of Nurses which was founded in 1913 by opening district centres, the first of which was opened at Kroonstad, followed shortly by one in Ladysmith, Natal.

In 1914 the Government contributed a sum of money to enable the order to establish a Non-White section. The work it accomplished over the years until its closure in 1960 included the inauguration of over 100 district nursing stations.

Other bodies whose work made a contribution to community health include:

- [ ] the Child Life Protection Society established in 1908, which in 1924 became the South African National Council for Child Welfare
- [ ] the South African Red Cross Society
- [ ] the South African National Council for the Blind
- [ ] the National Council for the Care of Cripples in South Africa, now the National Council for the Physically Disabled.

All these bodies and others had nurses attached to them to assist in the rendering of health care in the community according to their special aims and objectives. (Some information extracted from Searle 1965: ch 20.)

Role of missions

All the *mission hospitals* in the country developed some form of district nursing service in the areas they served, and in most cases they trained the indigenous population of the area as nurses and midwives to render such service. These nurses were especially well equipped to deal with community health problems and health education, belonging, as they did, to the communities they served.

The original Public Health Act was drawn up as a direct result of a disaster in community health, namely the 1918 influenza pandemic. Communities needed community care.

The district nursing service that originally developed to serve rural areas had also taken root in urban areas. These were aimed primarily at the extension of the care of the mother and child after the midwife and doctor had terminated their services, which was usually when the baby was ten days old.

The work of these 'health visitors' did a great deal to reduce maternal and child mortality. Health visiting *per se* grew out of a British concept according to which a person was employed to go from door to door in order to educate the poorer classes about hygiene and health as well as to uplift them socially and morally. When notification of births became compulsory and health visitors were required to visit each newborn baby and its mother in order to promote the health and welfare of both, it became necessary that some form of special training was instituted to prepare these workers for their task and courses were developed on a part-time basis at technical colleges.

It is from these beginnings that the current comprehensive courses have evolved.

Occupational health

As the country became more industrialised many firms, following world trends, began to pay more attention to the health of their workers, although the full importance of this aspect of community nursing has only received recognition with the publication of the report of the Erasmus Commission in 1976. The importance of occupational health does not yet receive the attention that it should. Many hospitals, for instance, which are large employers of personnel of all categories, do not have organised health services for all their employees. What service there is, is often haphazard and run along the lines of 'first-aid' for injuries or illness and little else. It is time that the health care delivery system became more organised in delivering comprehensive health care to its own personnel.

School nursing

In South Africa school nursing was established in 1914, and today the nurse bears the brunt of the school health service to Whites, Coloureds and Indians under the guidance of a handful of medical officers. The service to Blacks is only just being implemented.

The original concept of the 'public health nurse' or 'health visitor' being confined in her duties to immunisation and the prevention of communicable disease, environmental hygiene of the home and housing generally, to maternal and child care, the supervision of maternity homes and the provision of some form of health education has been broadened considerably. With modern medicine moving more and more into the community, the role of the community nurse has evolved and will continue to do so. There are no limits to her horizons.

The *Health Act*, 1977, (Act 63 of 1977) replaced the old and much amended *Public Health Act*, 1919 (Act 36 of 1919). In a guide to the Health Act, published by the then Department of Health, now the Department of National Health and Population Development, the following statements are made:

> As a result of the changing health situation in South Africa the consolidation, review and updating of the original Public Health Act, No. 36 of 1919, became a matter of urgency. The existing division of health functions between the Department of Health, provincial administrations and local authorities caused an escalating degree of inefficiency and overlapping of services. Consequently the health services could not develop in a co-ordinated manner and there was also a lack of uniform policy and implementation in respect of health and hospital services.
>
> The purpose of the Health Act is therefore to create by legislation, a blueprint for the rendering of health services by the three tiers of government and in so doing to regulate the functions between the authorities in the health field. Provision is made for the co-ordination of services and the determination of health policy on a national basis so that the

functions of the three health authorities can be adapted to utilize the available resources to the maximum and in so doing render the most effective health service to the population of South Africa (1977: 1).

No legislation is ever perfect. Times change, as do health needs, with advances in treatment and preventive measures. No doubt the new Act has flaws, but it has made many new developments, and especially coordination and cooperation, legally possible. Those who work in the national states have only one authority governing the rendering of health services, and thus 'the ideal of a comprehensive health service where equal attention is accorded to promotive, preventive, curative and rehabilitative health services has become a reality' (1977: 6). Many, however, work outside the national states, and the following quote from the same guide (1977: 19) states:

> The underlying philosophy of the Health Act No. 63 of 1977 is to create, by legislation, a blueprint for the present three tiers of Government to render health services in South Africa and to regulate the related functions between these authorities in the health field. In place of the rigidity of past health legislation a more flexible pattern is envisaged, in which powers, functions and duties of all the different authorities are reflected. Provision is also made for the co-ordination of services and the determining of health policy on a national basis so that the functions and duties of the different authorities can be adapted to utilize available resources to the maximum, making the most effective health service available to the public. The endeavours of the different authorities can thus be co-ordinated and directed to attain optimum results.

Practical implications of the Health Act for nursing may be found in Appendix B.

PRIMARY HEALTH CARE – THE ROLE OF THE NURSE

What is primary health care?

Primary health care, as the words imply, is the initial or *first* level of health care given to individuals needing or seeking that care. The whole population needs primary health care, for it is basic to attaining, retaining or regaining health, or making the best use of what health is left.

In a joint report by The World Health Organisation and the United Nations' Children's Fund (1978: 2) to the Alma-Ata conference in September 1978, the following definition was given:

> Primary Health Care is essential health care made universally accessible to individuals and families in the community by means acceptable to them, through their full participation and at a cost that the community and the country can afford. It forms an integral part, both of the country's health system of which it is the nucleus and of the overall social and economic development of the community.

It is thus not only curative, but preventive, promotive, rehabilitative and maintenance care.

Primary health care is also generally felt to be that form of health care given at the first point of contact of the client or patient with a member of the health care team. In the reality of the South African health care system, that health care team member is very often a nurse.

There are, however, many who are often forgotten as being health care workers. They are, however, absolutely essential to the provision of basic health services to all members of the community. They are an integral part of the health care system – health care in our present-day social system would be impossible without them.

Primary health care, if it is community-oriented and is to have community acceptance, as stated by the Alma-Ata conference (1978), must include:

- The provision of a *safe environment*, that is safe in terms of basic hygiene and housing, which includes safe water and food and safe disposal of excreta and other waste matter. This aims at preventing any first contact with other health care workers because of ill-health. It therefore provides primary care or basic care of first importance to health.
- *Adequate nutrition* for all.
- *Basic preventive health care* such as immunisation, antenatal and post-natal care, obstetric care, family planning and health education, as well as encouragement of individuals to accept responsibility for their own health and health practices.
- *Care for the aged, handicapped and chronic sick.*
- *Screening of persons* coming for specific health care because of a breakdown in health, and referral of those who need secondary level health care to more sophisticated services. This is followed by receiving them back after treatment, ongoing monitoring and care at the first basic or primary level once more.
- *The provision of services* needed to ensure that basic health care can reach all groups of the population and not only those people in, for example, upper income groups. This includes all members of groups such as mothers and children, toddlers and pre-school children, school children, adolescents, groups receiving tertiary education or post-school training, workers, the retired, the incapacitated and the aged.

A safe environment

Many persons are involved here, including those who may not be recognised by many readers as falling into the category of primary health care worker, but without whom our health services would be overburdened, if not brought to a complete standstill. Included are those who ensure a safe water supply for the community, food that is safe to eat, hygienic standards in public eating places and safe milk, as well as those who ensure adequate sewerage and waste disposal, those responsible for housing and slum prevention, and those who deal with the eradication of infection-carrying insects and rodents – all are primary health care workers.

The role of the nurse in this area is secondary and may be difficult for some to perceive. However, a community nurse can identify and point out problem areas such as a breakdown in services and the complete absence of the necessary services in some of the areas that she visits, or can observe and report conditions not conducive to healthy living in the community. Her role in this area may also include teaching people how to observe hygienic practices in child and home care that will ensure a safe environment for the family and thus for the community.

Adequate nutrition

Many agencies are concerned with this, as was only too evident in the recent drought during which the lack of water and famine caused so much ill-health. Specific workers concerned with nutrition, and thus with health, include those in agriculture, dieticians, paediatric specialists and other medical practitioners, as well as nutritionists generally.

The nurse, who so often has *continuous direct contact* with consumers of health care, can give patients or clients informed advice on basic nutritional needs. This is seen very clearly in the area of child health.

The nurse often has to act as the interpreter of instructions given by others. The patient, the mother of a child, the family member dealing with someone ill at home or recently discharged from hospital, will often ask the nurse for clarification of advice that has been given to them. The need for such explanation often arises as a result of the person concerned not wanting to appear ignorant to those originally giving the advice, or being too emotionally disturbed at the time to listen properly. Because the nurse has the opportunity for a more comfortable relationship with the client or patient than is often possible in the shorter doctor-patient contact, the person is more ready to ask the nurse if there is confusion in her mind about what was meant.

Basic preventive health care

Here the role of the nurse is more readily and generally understood.

Immunisation services are, on the whole, dependent on the nurse for their successful operation.

The *nurse-midwife*, particularly in the rural areas, gives ante-natal and post-natal care and delivers a large number of babies. She knows when she needs the medical man, especially when problems occur which are beyond her scope of practice and expertise.

The *family planning* services also rely on nurses to reach the people to a very large extent.

Health education, particularly at a personal, one-to-one level, and not just in the form of a 'dose of health education supplied by posters on clinic walls', as it has been described, can be given very effectively by the nurse. She does this by means of simple, appropriate advice, given at the right time, in the right place, in the applicable situation, using any teachable moment that may present itself. She also gives health education, unconsciously and by example, in her work and in community activities.

The nurse can *encourage* the individual to *accept responsibility* for his own health practices, often by subtle means, by reassurance and by tactfully pointing out alternatives. Again, the ready availability of a nurse in hospitals, clinics, in health care centres and in the community makes this possible.

Care of the aged, handicapped and chronic sick

This often falls fairly and squarely on the shoulders of the nurse. Physiotherapists and others also have an important part to play, as do medical practitioners who are on call in case of need. The monitoring of the chronic sick in old-age homes or at home is being carried out increasingly by nurses. This can also be regarded as basic or primary care.

Screening, treatment and referral

The modern professional nurse, who has completed at least four years of educational preparation, *can* and *is* being used to provide this service in many areas. The nurse involved in screening, treatment and referral poses no threat to anyone. Her function is to *assist* and *complement* and not to replace the medical practitioner in clinics, out-patient departments and other health services. A medical practitioner can practise only within the parameters of his education, training and expertise – with the professional nurse the situation is exactly the same.

Section 38(a) of the Nursing Amendment Act of September 1981 makes provision, in controlled situations, for the nurse to:

☐ physically examine any person

☐ diagnose any physical defect, illness or deficiency in any person

☐ keep prescribed medicines and supply, administer or prescribe them under the prescribed conditions

☐ promote family planning.

This may be done provided that the services of a medical practitioner or a pharmacist, as the circumstances may require, are not available. The way for the nurse to perform in a wider sphere has thus been legally opened.

We are all aware that there is a complete maldistribution of medical practitioners in the Republic of South Africa. Beaton and Bourne give the following figures: In 1975 the doctor to patient ratio was 1:875 in urban areas and 1:12 773 in rural areas – quite a contrast, you will agree. Further unpublished information from the same source states that 24% of the doctors in rural areas were not South African and that between 1975 and 1981 half of this 24% had disappeared from the registers of the South African Medical Council. This means that there would be little continuity of care and the possibility of doctors learning the language of the indigenous population would be very slim.

In clinics

In many outlying clinics with a large attendance of patients the nurse is the only health care worker available. Her medical cover often comes from a very long distance. Physical visits by doctors to these areas may occur only on a weekly, fortnightly, monthly or even longer spaced basis. Surely registered nurses with special in-service education would be able to give at least primary treatment?

The reality of the situation must never be forgotten. Those who have never been confronted with this type of situation may find it difficult to understand. Nurses in these situations carry the health services; without them there would be none.

In his 1983 report Dr Wessels, coordinator of primary health care services in the Eastern Cape and Border area, said that in the year 1982 the trained primary care sisters were involved in the management of nearly one million patient attendances in his area which, it must be pointed out, also included urban areas. In a personal discussion with the author he was quite emphatic that at least half a million of those treated would have received no care at all if it were not for the primary health care sisters. He stressed that such a practice required recent diplomates from a good educational system who had not yet become set in their ways or had time to become indoctrinated into the old system. They were specially selected for their knowledge, communication skills and adaptability and could, if given an in-service, updating and orientation period of about one month, function very effectively in such a service. He also stated that in the Transvaal, Baragwanath, with its eight primary health care clinics or polyclinics, handled between 60 000 and 70 000 patients a month and referred less than 4% of these to Baragwanath Hospital.

The primary health care sisters managed 70% of the patients alone – 30% were referred, half to the clinic's primary health care doctors and the rest to dentists, tuberculosis clinics, antenatal clinics, psychiatric clinics and others. In 1981 these clinics handled a total of 1 790 000 patients, who were seen by nurses only. Many more such clinics are envisaged in the future.

It is obvious that maximum use is being made of the potential of nurses in such circumstances. It is the stated policy of the authorities concerned with the provision of health care to all that the services will rely heavily on nurses in the future. There is no alternative.

As we have seen, primary health care also means a basic or first-level type of health care which, besides that provided in out-patient departments and clinics, is obtained in private practice. Is the maximum use being made of the registered nurse in this area?

In private practice

A medical practitioner is quite ready to accept the observations made by the nurse in the hospital situation, but sometimes seems reluctant to make similar use of nurses in consulting rooms. Here they are frequently used for clerical work such as booking appointments, recording visits, obtaining colleagues on the telephone and making tea! Could they not be better employed in taking basic health histories, doing preliminary examinations and carrying out certain tests?

It is not suggested that general practitioners spend less time with their patients – heaven forbid! However, armed with an essential health history and some preliminary observations and test results, a doctor could spend more time talking to the patient, confirming some problem area and deciding unhurriedly on an appropriate form of treatment based on a considered assessment of what he has before him, what he himself has observed and determined, and what his expertise tells him. It is the premise that, by appropriate use of the skills of the registered nurse, primary care in these circumstances could become more meaningful to patient and practitioner alike.

The registered nurse attached to a private practice could also be used to monitor patients at home and to do follow-up visits to assess the effectiveness of treatment, just as she does in a hospital or clinic. All this will be within the normal parameters of her professional practice. This type of practice could also lessen the burden of cost to the patient and add to patients' satisfaction with the care that they get.

Part-time nursing might bring many back into the profession for which they were trained but are not practising.

Provision of services needed

The provision of services for basic health care to reach all groups of the population is the final element of primary health care. Many people in the community buy health services, either in their private capacity or through their medical aid schemes. For the most part these people have services available if they become ill and also have access to preventive services.

However, there are numerous members of the population of the Republic of South Africa who do not have access to medical aid schemes and cannot afford to buy services. They would not think of preventive services in any case, except perhaps compulsory immunisation for children, and often not even this. It is obvious that if primary care services are to be provided in all areas such as child health care, occupational health care and health care for students, trainees, the handicapped and senior citizens, then the services of the nurse must be used extensively.

Most of our school health services operate almost exclusively on nursing personnel. Nurses are also being used in psychiatric services, in oncology services, in genetic services and in primary midwifery services. All of them provide basic, first-line or primary health care.

The registered nurse follows a controlled educational programme that is constantly undergoing review and revision to meet the changing needs of the times. Nurses form by far the largest group of professional workers in the health field. They are expected to exercise educated judgement in their work. The attitude of those who do make full use of the services of nurses is not in question, but the attitude of those who employ nurses but do not use them optimally does require examination.

The best possible care of patients and clients is the aim of all members of the health care team. Improving the quality of that care by utilising the registered nurse, teaching her skills that she can use but may not yet have acquired, and accepting her as a person able to make a valuable contribution in the team approach to patient care can only be of benefit to all.

From what has been said it would appear that *primary health care* is given by members of the community and by health care professionals, including medical practitioners, pharmacists, dieticians and members of the supplementary health professions, as well as by social workers. However, the nurse could be the core figure in the rendering of primary health care because of the number of nurses available, the initimacy of the nurse's continuous contact with members of the community, well and ill, and her latent expertise which, it has been proved, can be evolved to meet specific needs in a given situation in many different areas.

* * * * *

In 1986 the Government published new thoughts on health care entitled 'A new dispensation: health services for South Africa'. This spells out a National Health Plan and Policy that will give direction to the development of health services in the future. For details see Appendix C.

PRIVATISATION

The government of the day has committed itself to a policy of privatisation. This includes health care services in general and hospitalisation in particular.

The health care in the private sector has depended on health care personnel trained largely by the public sector, and there is a considerable reservoir of expertise and skill that is not used for the education and training of health personnel at present. It is felt that the private sector should use its facilities and personnel to make a contribution to the preparation of health personnel as a whole. The education and training of nurses, who form the largest single group of health care workers, is neglected. Their preparation, especially that of the sub-professional categories, has been started in some areas, but this will have to be expanded considerably as privatisation of health care increases so that the personnel needed for health care in the country at large can be provided. Education and training of nurses for registration as well as for post-registration specialisation must be undertaken by the private sector. This is an area for future development.

SPECIALISATION IN NURSING

A section has already been devoted to the evolving role of the nurse, but it was more concerned with changes in the role and function of nurses in general. This section will look at the various specialist fields that have developed in the practice of the art and science of nursing. Medical science has long felt the need for specialisation and it is no accident that nursing, the sister profession of medicine, has developed similar needs.

By the middle of the seventeenth century medical thought was influenced by the scientific approach of the times, which paved the way for great discoveries and victories over many diseases. The eighteenth century saw the establishment of the teaching of anatomy at medical schools. Percussion as a diagnostic technique was founded by Auenbrugger and pathology as a separate study owes its origins to Morgagni.

Jenner discovered vaccination, but it was the modern period, starting after the French Revolution, that was to bring the most dramatic changes. These remarkable scientific discoveries included many in the fields of chemistry and biochemistry. The number of discoveries in the scientific field became so large and so diverse that medical knowledge split into several distinct branches and specialisation was born. This specialisation has become more and more varied, so that new specialist fields appear with increasing rapidity. Some of the discoveries that led to specialisation in medicine were the following:

- The discovery of anaesthesia, from which the specialist *anaesthetist* has evolved
- Developments in the fields of vaccination and immunisation generally, from the study of which has evolved the *immunologist*
- Revolutionary developments in microbiology, giving us the *microbiologist*
- The discovery of X-rays and radium, which led not only to increased diagnostic potential but to radiotherapy, including the use of radioactive isotopes, etc, leading to specialisation in this field
- Discoveries of new drugs – an ongoing process that has given us our specialist *pharmacologists*
- Advances in the field of technology and biomedical engineering; computer diagnosis, heart-lung machines, electronic monitors and defibrillators; and advances in aerospace medicine and renal dialysis – all have produced their crop of specialists, experts in their special fields.

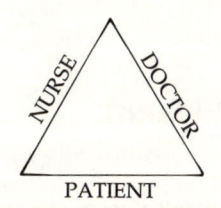

Improved diagnostic tools and techniques have greatly increased man's knowledge and people have begun specialisation in many other areas. No one can know all about everything. Therefore physicians have concentrated their energies on acquiring as much knowledge about a particular field as is humanly practicable. The practice of medicine is no longer confined to the old established triad:

The patient – or the client, if he is a well person and the ultimate aim is to keep him so – is still there. The single doctor or medical man has been replaced by a team of doctors, technicians and paramedical workers. The nurse has also developed a multi-disciplinary approach. The advent of specialisation in medicine has produced, in addition to the above-mentioned, the physician specialist, the general surgeon specialist, the orthopaedic specialist, the urologist, the otorhinolaryngologist, the obstetrician-gynaecologist, the plastic surgeon, the maxillo-facial specialist, the neuro-surgeon, the thoracic surgeon, the ophthalmologist, the neurologist, the psychiatrist, the gerontologist, the paediatrician, the oncologist, the geneticist, the pathologist and the endocrinologist.

This list is by no means complete and is constantly receiving additions. In the fields related to medicine specialist developments have resulted in physiotherapists, occupational therapists, pharmacists, biochemists, laboratory technicians, machine technicians, optometrists and dieticians and diet therapists.

With all this development in medicine and its related disciplines, the development of the specialist nurse was inevitable. While the basic disciplines of nursing are considered to be general clinical nursing, midwifery and psychiatric nursing, with community nursing now becoming a basic discipline it is inevitable that the nurse working in close contact with the medical specialist will develop an expertise that makes her a specialist in her own right.

Many of these specialised directions have been recognised by the creation of a specific post-basic course. These have proliferated. Some are recognised by certification and registration, others are post-basic in-service courses. At the moment there is a great need for the integration of common core material in many post-basic courses so that time and money-consuming repetition can be avoided. The South African Nursing Council is currently giving attention to this matter. Basic courses also require coordination and more integration so that specialisation can be built on foundations that are soundly laid. Repetitive work kills initiative.

At present the following official post-registration courses are available in the Republic of South Africa:

- opthalmic nursing science
- orthopaedic nursing science
- paediatric nursing science
- operating theatre nursing science
- intensive nursing science
- nursing administration
- nursing education
- psychiatric nurse instruction
- geriatric nursing science
- oncology nursing science
- clinical nursing science, health assessment, treatment and care.

There are also advanced courses in disciplines such as advanced midwifery and neonatal nursing science, advanced psychiatric nursing science and advanced paediatric and neonatal nursing science.

In addition, there are non-official in-service courses such as the paediatric nurse practitioner course offered in the Cape. At the same time clinical specialisation has grown up in nursing in renal care units, with stomatherapists and many others. The needs of most of these can be met by in-service programmes to fill gaps or to teach new skills, although some become full courses as things develop. Post-registration certificate courses in occupational health nursing, renal nursing, stoma care nursing, spinal injury nursing and intensive neonatal nursing are also available.

The present diversity in the work of the nurse can only increase and she must see this as a natural development wherever her services are needed to provide care for the sick. The nurse has accepted the challenge of modern medicine and equipped herself to meet changed circumstances, and she must continue to do this. Highly skilled, carefully educated and, in many instances, highly specialised nurses capable of taking their places alongside the other members of the therapeutic team to provide total health care must constantly be developed.

The specialist nurse, as a nurse consultant to her less experienced colleagues, as a leader and as a teacher is here to stay. As long as she does not let her newly developed technical skill make her forget the essential humanness of those for whom she is caring she will fulfil the highest traditions of her profession, no matter what direction her specialisation takes.

The nurse specialist in the clinical field could be available throughout the hospital. She would belong to a special medical field. She would not supplant the ward sister (professional nurse in charge of a ward), but would assist her. She would assist the generalist, the ward sister, in the same way that the medical specialist assists the general practitioner. She would be specialist in a technological sense, because she would have to keep abreast of new developments in her field. She would act as a consultant and be seen as such by her nursing colleagues. She would not carry out the specialist nursing programme herself, but teach her colleagues and students to give the expert care of which she is master. In her specialist capacity she would teach, ascertain competence, check standards and move on. She would be a 'troubleshooter' *par excellence*, for, by the very nature of her work, she would deal with problem areas and bring her expertise to bear in solving such problems.

There is a great future for specialisation in nursing, as in any other field, provided it is handled carefully and that the specialists, remaining true nurses, keep the highest ideals of their profession always before them.

4 The profession of nursing

Many of the ideas expressed in this chapter originated out of lectures given by Professor C Searle which the author attended while studying for the MCur (Nursing Education) at the University of Pretoria. (The degree was awarded in March 1971.) Ideas were also crystallised during discussions, seminars and assignments which were part of this study.

PROFESSIONALISM

A great deal has been written about professions and professionalism, but confusion still exists in the minds of many people. Originally, professions were seen as the services provided to people by the church. These included health care, teaching, welfare work and law.

Later, universities took over the function of training people for the professions. Public services such as welfare of the sick poor became the responsibility of secular organisations.

Protestantism changed the emphasis to family care for those who needed such services. Originally people 'professed' belief in a religion. Often there was a feeling of divine calling. On taking her vows the nun made her 'profession'. With the passage of time this meaning has broadened and changed, but a professional occupation still retains certain characteristics. These signify that a profession is more than merely an occupation or a sphere of work by means of which one earns one's daily bread.

The fact that a profession is more than a means of obtaining a livelihood does not mean that one cannot receive payment for professional work, or that it should not be adequately rewarded in monetary terms. Since Flexner first identified the criteria in terms of which he judged whether medicine was a profession or not, many other authorities have identified criteria in terms of which a profession should be measured, including Carr-Saunders & Wilson (1933) and Lysaught (1970).

What makes a profession different from a job may be summarised as follows:

A profession is characterised by:
- a large body of specialised theory with well-developed technical skills based on this theory

- ☐ the use of theory from the sciences and other fields of learning are relevant to its practice
- ☐ a long period of specialised preparation at a recognised educational institution
- ☐ the testing of professional competence before admission to the ranks of the profession
- ☐ some recognised form of registration and licence to practice
- ☐ self-organisation leading to the formation of a professional association and a self-governing body which controls professional standards
- ☐ ethical control of professional conduct by members of the profession
- ☐ a motive of service based on the client's needs for professional assistance, irrespective of his ability to pay for services rendered – the welfare of the client is the overriding consideration
- ☐ a high degree of accountability for professional acts, to the public, the client and the employing body and other members of the profession
- ☐ a feeling of exclusiveness
- ☐ a recognised status in law
- ☐ a high social status and considerable social power
- ☐ the performance of activities based on an understanding of what is involved in these activities so that the results of acts or omissions can be predicted. The individual profession must thus decide for itself which subjects should be studied in its educational programme in order that this understanding may be achieved
- ☐ constant critical analysis of its activities leading to the modification of practice in the light of this analysis. Thus a profession is never static, but subject to constant change and development. This leads to the discarding of what is no longer relevant in favour of what is of more use in carrying out the activities related to the nature of the occupation
- ☐ the ability of its members to select in a responsible manner the activities that are of intrinsic importance to its practice. These activities must also be realistically attainable by the members of the profession
- ☐ the individual member being allowed the maximum use of discretion and initiative in practice. Independent functions and accountability for their performance are inherent
- ☐ the obligation of members to use their best endeavours at all times in meeting the needs of clients
- ☐ a continuous striving for excellence – competence is not enough.

These criteria, compiled from the opinions of authoritative writers, are those in terms of which occupations can be measured to determine whether they qualify for rating as professions.

There are differences of opinion among writers on this subject. Some have a much narrower concept of a profession, requiring, among other things, university education, self-employment and complete independence in the practice of the profession.

If these limited criteria were to be applied, no one who was not prepared for practice by university education would qualify to be called a professional person. The practitioners of many occupations that are universally regarded as professions obtain their qualifications by means of other forms of education such as qualifying associations. These professional practitioners include barristers, medical specialists and clergymen educated at theological seminaries.

The requirement that professionals must be self-employed is also invalid. Many established professions have practising members who are not self-employed, but work for a salary. This group includes ministers of religion, who receive a stipend and members of the legal profession, who are extensively employed in industry and commerce, in various forms of public service and in military service. They do not become non-professionals because they are paid a salary. A judge is paid a fixed salary by the state. Medical men are often in the employ of the state health services, provincial or local authorities, industry or commerce and receive a salary in payment for their services.

The requirement that a professional must have complete independence of practice can also be challenged. Any professional, irrespective of whether he is paid a salary, is responsible for his own professional acts. He cannot ignore this aspect of his work, which makes him an independent practitioner without him having to set up and run his own practice.

Nursing as a profession

The vocation of nursing, which is as old as man himself, has passed through many more changes than most other occupations. Until comparatively recently, the only nursing to which the title profession could justifiably have been appended was that inspired by religious or at least charitable motives. This led to nurses in the religious orders being called to a life devoted to the care of the sick.

Those who were charitably disposed, although not necessarily members of religious orders, also cared for the sick as a philanthropic act, but the majority of sufferers were out of reach of these people and had to rely on family, friends or other persons. After the collapse of many religious orders that followed the reformation, no lay orders replaced the women to whom devoted service to the sick was a tradition. For three centuries nursing as a profession largely disappeared in the West.

Without the religious conviction that caring for the sick was a Christian duty, the caring for the sick and forlorn poor became a sordid chore fit only for those on the lowest rung of the social scale, who were often drunken, destitute widows.

The Quaker influence in the nineteenth century did something to restore the balance, making caring for the sick and poor a valued Christian virtue once more. In 1840 Elizabeth Fry influenced the founding of an institute of nursing which trained nurses. Interest in this matter began to be felt in other circles, which was in keeping with the generally felt need for social reform. St John's House, where nurses were trained for Kings College Hospital, was founded in 1848. However, it is due to the endeavours of Florence Nightingale that nursing began the long road back to the professional status that it enjoys today.

In the Republic of South Africa it can be clearly demonstrated that nursing has achieved the recognition and status of a profession. Before discussing the rights and obligations that nurses in this country have because of this professional status, each criterion for a profession will be discussed separately and the way in which nursing in South Africa measures up to the stated criteria will be demonstrated.

Criterion 1 – A profession is characterised by a large body of specialised theory with well-developed technical skills based on this theory

Nursing has a body of specialised knowledge or theory based on the application of the nursing process to the unique function that the nurse fulfils. Modern nursing is a scientific process consisting of essential phases that occur in sequence and are all necessary. These segmental phases form the nursing process.

Assessment of the situation

The nurse must be able to make all the relevant observations of the patient or client for whom she has to care, whether in the preventive, promotive or rehabilitative field of her work, with intelligent judgement and must be able to synthesize this information in order to carry out the next phase of the sequence. She must be able to diagnose the nursing needs that she as a nurse can meet independently and the need for referral of the client to other members of the health team. It follows that a nurse requires a high degree of specialised theoretical knowledge to be able to exercise the required intelligent judgement, synthesis of information and diagnosis of nursing or referral needs.

Planning a course of action

Having assessed the situation and determined the needs, the nurse must propose a course of action. This may necessitate immediate and swift emergency action. It entails the establishment of priorities, that is deciding what requires immediate action and what can wait, in fact what should wait. This planning must be both short and long term. The proposed plan of action must be flexible so that it can be changed to meet any emergency.

Application of the plan of action

When the situation has been assessed and the course of action planned, the nurse must put her plan of action into effect, either by acting herself or by delegating the carefully delineated tasks to those working with her. Again this requires knowledge and technical skill based on that knowledge. The technical skill that can be expected of other categories of workers is part of the knowledge the nurse must have. These other categories may include the assistant nurse who, because of her limited knowledge and preparation, is a non-professional member of the nursing team and works under direct or indirect supervision of the professional who has the necessary preparation and knowledge.

Concurrent and retrospective appraisal

This entails deciding whether the action or actions taken are having the desired effect, in other words whether the patient or client, or the community, is reacting as anticipated to the nursing action. If not, re-evaluation of the situation, an amended plan of action, application of the amended plan and reappraisal become necessary. Retrospective appraisal helps to determine past deficiencies and should lead to improvements in the evaluation of any situation, better future plans of action, improvement in the application of the plan of action and more competent future appraisal. It is obvious that up-to-date specialised knowledge is necessary. No appraisal of results can occur without this.

Recording

Records of the nurse's assessment and of the action taken, as well as of the outcome of this action, are necessary to provide evidence that the nurse has given care for which she, as a professional person, is accountable. Records also help in appraisal, in the determination of deficiencies and in the planning of improved future care. If it is not based on sound specialised knowledge, record-keeping can be meaningless and valueless. Technical skill is necessary at all phases of the nursing process, but it is imperative that this technical skill keeps abreast of modern trends. This entails continous additions to the store of specialised theory necessary for entry into the profession.

Criterion 2 – A profession is characterised by the use of theory from the sciences and other fields of learning relevant to its practice

The specialised knowledge and skills upon which the nursing profession in South Africa bases its theory are derived from the biological, physical, medical and social sciences, from philosophy, from the accumulation of nursing knowledge gained from the practice of nursing throughout the ages, and from the legal and ethical concepts upon which any profession rests. Any syllabus laid down for the education of the neophyte professional nurse contains courses such as applied physical science and chemistry, anatomy and physiology, the ethos of the profession, microbiology, pharmacology and pathology, nursing art and science, sociology and social work, psychology and the science of preventive and promotive health. Syllabusses are revised from time to time in order to keep up with modern knowledge. This meets the requirements for criterion 2.

Criterion 3 – A profession is characterised by a long period of specialised preparation at a recognised educational institution

Preparation for professional nursing in South Africa requires a minimum of four years' education at diploma level before registration, midwifery, psychiatric nursing science and community nursing science being included. Degree preparation at university level leading to the same registrations takes from four to four-and-a-half years. The post-basic diplomas and degrees available for specialisation in a branch of nursing require one to three years of study.

Thus the criterion of a long period of preparation is met. The diploma courses are offered at colleges of nursing in association with universities, and have to be officially recognised by the South African Nursing Council, which is the registration body. Post-basic diplomas are offered at universities, nursing colleges, hospitals and some technikons (the diploma in community nursing). Thus the second part of criterion 3 is met.

Criterion 4 – A profession is characterised by the testing of professional competence before admission to the ranks of the profession

Again the South African nursing profession meets this criterion. Before any diploma or degree may be registered as a nursing qualification the neophyte has to pass professional examinations. Colleges in cooperation with universities conduct their own examinations moderated by the university concerned.

For the most part, the examiners come from the peer group. Qualified nurses act as examiners. In some instances medical practitioners or other professional experts also participate. Universities set and control their own examinations, although the syllabusses of courses, the composition of curricula and the arrangement for practica during the course have to be approved by the South African Nursing Council as well. The nursing education offered by universities is also subject to Nursing Council inspection, as is that offered by nursing colleges in conjunction with hospitals.

Post-basic diploma courses also have to be approved for registration by the South African Nursing Council, which also controls and conducts examinations. Some post-basic diploma courses are examined by the Department of National Education, while those offered by universities are examined by the university concerned. Nursing examinations conducted by universities are subject to the same rules and procedures as examinations in any other university subject.

Proof of the education undergone is also a prerequisite for registration. This control of examinations and of admission to the register is a guarantee to the public that anyone claiming to be a registered nurse has attained a certain standard approved by the profession. It is a safeguard of the rights of the clients entrusted to the care of nurses.

Criterion 5 – A profession is characterised by some recognised form of registration and licence to practice

It has already been stated that the South African Nursing Council is the registering body, its main function being the maintenance of registers of various categories of nurses and rolls of other categories.

Current registration is a requirement for practice. A registered professional nurse is admitted to the register in South Africa after having undergone the required period and type of education and passed the examinations.

The register of nurses in South Africa is a living one, the registered nurse being required to renew her licence to practise every year by payment of a stipulated fee. The name of a registered nurse may be removed from the register for non-payment of the annual fee or for contravention of the ethical code after a disciplinary inquiry has established guilt and laid down the penalty. A name may also be voluntarily removed from the register if a nurse no longer wishes to practise. It must be emphasised that once a nurse's name has been removed from the register for any reason whatsoever it is a criminal offence if she uses the title registered nurse or practises nursing for gain in any capacity whatsoever. Registration of nursing qualifications by the South African Nursing Council is laid down as a function of the Council by the Nursing Act.

The South African Nursing Council is responsible for prescribing requirements for admission to nursing education, prescribing syllabusses, approving and inspecting schools of nursing, examinations of competence and registration of qualifications. Thus the fifth criterion is met.

Criterion 6 – A profession is characterised by self-organisation leading to the formation of a professional association and a self-governing body which controls professional standards

The members of a profession decide among themselves how their profession will function. They lay down the ethical codes, standards, admission requirements and other matters pertaining to the practice of the profession. This control by the profession itself is jealously guarded. The self-governing aspect of a profession is regulated by statute.

In 1891 the seal of professionalism was firmly stamped on the nursing profession with the registration of the first professional nurse in Southern Africa, indeed, the first registration of a nurse in the world. Since then professional nurses have successfully organised and developed the profession.

The nursing profession in South Africa has its self-governing functions laid down by Act of Parliament, that is the Nursing Act, which was first passed in 1944, when a dedicated body of trained nurses who had formed the South African Trained Nurses' Association saw the danger of the trade union movement to professionalism in nursing and took action to ensure the future of the profession in South Africa. The Nursing Act of 1944 was replaced by Act No 50 of 1978 and amended by Act 71 of 1981.

The 1944 Act made provision for the formation of two statutory bodies namely the South African Nursing Council, a registering authority with clearly outlined powers and functions, and the South African Nursing Association, a professional association of nurses. These two bodies are discussed in detail later in the text.

Criterion 7 – A profession is characterised by ethical control of professional conduct by its own members

Here again the nursing profession meets the criterion. Nurses in this country are subject to an ethical code laid down by members of the profession. The regulation of ethical practice is the function of the South African Nursing Council. Regulations, promulgated by the Department of National Health and Population Development, are drawn up for the conditions under which various categories of nurses may practise their profession. These regulations are subject to review and amendment as conditions change.

Suspected or reported deviations from the ethical code are investigated and a disciplinary inquiry is held where necessary. The nurse is tried by a committee of peers and is given the opportunity of defending herself personally or by means of legal representation if she wishes to do so. The committee determines the guilt or otherwise of the person charged. If she is found guilty, the various penalties that may be imposed are laid down. These include reprimand, reprimand and caution, suspension of name from the register or roll for a specific period, removal of name from the register or roll and, in the case of students, lengthening of the period of training.

Sentence passed has to be confirmed by the full Council.

Thus the ethical control of nursing in South Africa rests firmly in the hands of the profession under delegated responsibility from Parliament.

Criterion 8 – A profession is characterised by a motive of service, based on the needs of the client for professional assistance, irrespective of his ability to pay for services rendered. The welfare of the client is the overriding consideration

Of course, this criterion does not imply that payment cannot be asked or accepted for professional service, but simply that where a need exists and there is no possibility of payment the service cannot be denied. This does not mean that nurses should be exploited. Just as they recognise the human dignity and rights of others, so their human dignity and rights as professional people must be recognised. The foundation of nursing rests on a human need, the need for health and for care when health is impaired.

Nursing, one of the oldest vocations, has passed through its bleak periods. In the past it was inspired by religious, or at least philanthropic, motives. When these motives ceased to exist nursing went through its own dark ages. The light of true nursing was kept alive in some measure by the care given by religious institutions, but its resurgence was due to people such as Elizabeth Fry and Florence Nightingale. The true spirit of nursing still shines brightly in a troubled world.

The practice of the profession of nursing has undergone profound changes so that today the professional nurse receives adequate remuneration for nursing services and has opportunities to further her nursing education and at the same time to lead a normal social life as a member of the community. The underlying spirit of service has not disappeared. Nursing is a caring profession. Of all the members of the health team the nurse has the closest and most continuous contact with the client or patient, whatever the sphere in which she is functioning. Few other health workers have the opportunity to build up such a relationship of trust with the client. The caring function of the nurse is an independent function. It entails giving service based on needs, service over and above anything that can be rewarded in monetary terms. Without this service motive, nursing as we understand it cannot exist. Technical skill may be employed and applied, but without the spirit of caring and service this becomes the work of a technician, a mechanical action and not nursing.

Nursing leaders in South Africa are constantly stating this fact. This philosophy is part of every educational programme for the preparation of the professional nurse practitioner. As long as this service motive is held high by all professional nurses, then this eighth criterion is also met.

Criterion 9 – A profession is characterised by a high degree of accountability for professional acts to the public, the client and the employing body and other members of the profession

It has already been shown how the ethical code of the nursing profession is upheld in the Republic of South Africa. It must be stressed that the nurse is responsible for her own professional acts and omissions. A nurse is accountable for professional competence, judgement and action. Treatment can be prescribed for a patient, but the manner in which the nurse carries out the treatment is her individual responsibility. Of course, this applies to all categories of nurses.

A nurse has a duty to her client, to the public, to her employing body and to the other members of the profession to maintain competence, to keep up to date, to preserve the rights and human dignity of others and to practise the profession of nursing faithfully, within the provisions of the Act and the regulations promulgated under it. Personal integrity, the exercise of independent judgement in professional action and an awareness that by her actions she attaches a label to the nursing profession as a whole, helps to foster in the nurse the sense of responsibility and the recognition of accountability that are necessary for meeting this criterion.

South African professional nurses constantly strive to meet this most exacting requirement. They recognise their responsibility to those they serve, to those who work with them in the health team and to those for whom they work. They know that they are accountable for their professional acts and equally accountable for professional omissions and thus they meet the requirements of criterion 9.

Criterion 10 – A profession is characterised by a feeling of exclusiveness

This criterion is easily understood. A member of a profession has a sense of belonging to a group different from other groups. By the very actions of prescribing admission requirements, registration and licence to practise, the profession defines its own exclusivity. Thus medical doctors feel a common bond, as do sociologists, members of the legal profession, members of the teaching profession and architects. By virtue of their profession and the limitation of membership imposed by the peer group, they are different from others. The same can be said of professional nurses. They belong to an exclusive body of professional people.

Criterion 11 – A profession is characterised by a recognised status in law

In order to attain the status of a profession an occupation has to be recognised by the Parliament of the land, which accords members of the profession rights and privileges, provides for registration of members and lays down procedures for the peer-group control of the profession which include admission requirements, professional standards and ethical control. Seeing that the profession of nursing in South Africa is regulated by Act of Parliament, it meets this criterion.

Criterion 12 – A profession is characterised by high social status and considerable social power

Any recognised profession, because of its service motive, achieves public recognition, respect, and therefore a high social status. This status is ascribed by virtue of membership of the profession as such, and not as a result of material or other considerations. Services which meet human needs are highly valued by society. Those who supply these services are also highly valued and their social status is enhanced. A position of mutual trust and respect is built up. Adherence to a code of professional conduct is expected. The public depends on professional people to act in a responsible manner, and those who do so acquire considerable social power. Threats and demonstrations are not expected from professional people, nor are strikes. Disputes are handled by consultation and arbitration.

The nursing profession in South Africa meets these requirements. Members are not prepared to use the lives of patients as a bargaining instrument. What they have gained for themselves in the way of improvements in service conditions and privileges and in increased educational facilities to improve their professional competence has been gained by negotiation. This is recognised by the community in the form of social status accorded to members of the profession. With the social power that they wield nurses are constantly battling for improved health facilities for the community and for health education for all members of the population.

The nursing profession performs an important social function in that it serves as the vital link between the products of the scientific laboratory and the human being to whom the laboratory discoveries are applied. Ultimately it is the nurse who, because she has worked with persons requiring care and for their benefit, has knowledge acquired through close contact with people in their homes, in clinics, in industry, in the community and in the hospital which enables her to press for change.

The power to initiate changes in the social conditions that contribute to ill-health lies in the hands of the nurse. In South Africa, she uses this power for the common good.

Criterion 13 – A profession is characterised by the performance of activities based on an understanding of what is involved in these activities so that results of acts or omissions can be predicted. The individual profession must thus decide for itself which subjects should be studied in its educational programme in order that this understanding may be achieved

It has already been pointed out that the nurse is accountable for her acts or omissions. If she is to be capable of exercising considered judgement based on sound scientific knowledge, her educational programme will have to be broadly based. The subjects that nurses in South Africa have to study are laid down by the South African Nursing Council, that is by members of the profession itself. These are constantly under review and are amended as required in the light of the latest medical and scientific knowledge and to meet the needs of the evolving role of the nurse. Thus criterion 13 is also met.

Criterion 14 – A profession is characterised by constant critical analysis of its activities leading to the modification of practice in the light of this analysis. Thus a profession is never static, but subject to constant change and development. This leads to the discarding of what is no longer relevant in favour of what is of more use in the carrying out of the activities related to the nature of the occupation

Nursing activities in South Africa are constantly under review, and it is necessary only to think back over the last two decades to realise what significant developments have taken place. Despite the resistance to change evident among some members of the profession, old methods have been discarded and replaced by new ones, often initiated by nurses with vision and innovative ability. Thus this criterion is also met.

Criterion 15 – A profession is characterised by the ability of its members to select, in a responsible manner, the activities that are of intrinsic importance to its practice. These activities must also be realistically attainable by the members of the profession

Although this criterion ties in with criterion 14, it goes a step further in that nurses have been responsible enough to see their evolving role and have taken steps to ensure that activities that were formerly considered to fall outside their sphere of work and that they perform with competence are accepted as part of their professional practice. In this acceptance they have also been responsible enough to recognise where new skills must be learned; and they have taken steps to make good their shortcomings as individuals and those of the personnel for whom they are responsible. The necessary skills training has also been incorporated in their basic educational programme.

Criterion 16 – A profession is characterised by the individual member being allowed the maximum use of discretion and initiative in practice. Independent functions and accountability for their performance are inherent

Although this criterion ties in with criterion 9, it goes even further. It recognises that the nurse has many independent functions and uses her own discretion and initiative in the performance of her professional acts. She is in charge of the nursing care of the patients or clients committed to her care. She must use her discretion, based on up-to-date knowledge, and her initiative when making a nursing diagnosis and planning and implementing care. True, she is accountable for her independent acts, but as a professional nurse she must be prepared to use her discretion and initiative. If she does not do so, but waits for 'orders' or instructions, her lack of action is unprofessional.

Criterion 17 – A profession is characterised by the obligation of members to use their best endeavours at all times in meeting the needs of clients

Nurses in South Africa, as well as elsewhere, are expected to give of their best at all times. The welfare of patients or clients is entrusted to them. A patient's life may depend on the person caring for him. If that care is given in an inefficient way, if the nurse is unreliable or careless, or if her mind is on other matters she will not use her endeavours to the utmost and will fail to fulfil this obligation. She will be guilty of transgressing an unwritten ethical code. Because the nursing profession in South Africa cherishes the ideal of members giving of their best at all times in the service of patients or clients, it also meets this criterion.

Criterion 18 – A profession is characterised by a continuous striving for excellence – competence is not enough

The nurse strives to meet this criterion by concurrent self-evaluation, evaluation of the care given by those over whom she has jurisdiction and insistence on quality care for patients. The existence of many updating in-service education courses, the eagerness with which continuing nursing education programmes are received and the constant endeavours of many nurses in this country to gain new knowledge is further evidence of the professional status of nursing.

* * *

Nursing in South Africa meets all the criteria of a profession. It is up to the members of the profession to see themselves in this light.

A registered nurse is a professional person with responsibilities as well as rights because of her acceptance of her professional role. She must therefore have the utmost regard for her profession and its ethical code. She must hold its image high and never forget the service motive upon which her existence as a professional person is based. She must guard her professional standing against inroads by other groups. She has a unique position in service to the community. The continuity and closeness of her association with her clients, both those who are ill and need her services to help them in the struggle to combat illness and regain health and those who are striving to prevent ill-health in themselves and the members of their families, place the nurse in a position of trust. She must maintain her competence and increase it, at all times give of her best in the performance of her professional duties, and keep the service motive always before her.

A knowledge of what constitutes a profession and of the concept of professionalism related to her own sphere of activity should help to instil in the nurse a sense of pride in the profession that will contribute to quality patient care.

COMPOSITION OF THE NURSING PROFESSION IN SOUTH AFRICA

The nursing profession in South Africa is composed of members of various races, mostly, although not always, engaged in the service of their own people. It is composed of men and women of all ages. The number of men who are nurses is very small in proportion to the number of women, but they nevertheless play an important role in the profession, especially in some health services to which they are ideally suited.

The members of the profession include a large number of married women. These women tend to marry and then work until their first babies are due. Many return to work when their babies are quite young, and it is to cater for this group that many hospitals have crèche facilities. Others complete their families of two or three children and return to work only after the youngest goes to school or at least nursery school. It is for this group that in-service updating programmes are essential. Without such programmes valuable practitioners are lost to nursing due to their fears that changes will have taken place during the time that they were not actively nursing. In a predominantly female profession this aspect merits serious consideration by all employers of nurses.

Today the profession includes the following categories of registered nurses (it will be seen that many are registered in more than one capacity):
☐ Registered general nurses
☐ Registered general nurses and midwives
☐ Registered psychiatric nurses
☐ Registered psychiatric nurses and midwives
☐ Registered general nurses and psychiatric nurses
☐ Registered general nurses, midwives, and psychiatric nurses
☐ Registered general nurses, midwives, psychiatric nurses and community nurses.

It is not advisable to give detailed figures here since they need constant updating. Suffice it to say that the above categories as at 31 December 1986 made up a total of 64 917 persons, of whom 26 969 were Black, 5 737 Coloured, 1 386 Indian, and 30 825 White (SANC statistics).

It is impossible to work out a ratio of registered nurses to the various race groups, since there are many examples of people serving an ethnic group different from their own.

The nursing profession in South Africa also includes various categories of students who are registered nurses in embryo.

Apart from the professional category of registered nurses, there is the sub-professional group consisting of enrolled nurses and pupil enrolled nurses. The number of enrolled persons as at 31 December 1986 totalled 23 924, of whom 15 574 were Black, 3 856 Coloured, 490 Indian and 4 004 White (SANC statistics).

Besides this there are the non-professional group of enrolled nursing assistants. The total number as at 31 December 1986 was 42 155, of whom 25 046 were Black, 7 776 Coloured, 593 Indian and 8 740 White.

The preparation and scope of practice of enrolled categories is presently under review. Students should be alert to changes that may result.

The number of registered nurses holding post-basic qualifications is also important when the composition of the profession is considered. Many registered nurses, besides maintaining one or more basic registrations, are also registered in more than one capacity obtained at post-basic level. Thus in December 1986 there were the following registrations of post-basic qualifications (groups in which numbers were very small are omitted):

Capacities	Number of persons as at 31/12/86				
	Total	White	Coloured	Indian	Black
Degree/Diploma					
Nurse Educator (Tutor)	2 068	1 489	144	37	698
Nurse Administrator	2 159	1 173	106	32	848
Diplomas					
Clinical Care, Administration and Instruction	1 618	493	217	26	882
Clinical Nursing Science, Health Assessment, Treatment and Care	475	13	4	10	448
Community Nursing Science	5 328	2 762	538	156	1 872
Intensive Nursing Science	1 665	992	167	35	471
Operating Theatre Nursing Science	2 824	1 636	146	35	907
Ophthalmic Nursing Science	318	36	12	9	261
Orthopaedic Nursing Science	830	321	71	9	429
Paediatric Nursing Science	1 488	598	174	21	695
Certificates					
Mothercraft	430	280	45	11	94
Obstetric Analgesia and Recuscitation	394	334	4	5	51
Occupational Health Nursing	388	328	17	6	37

It is important that anyone reading these figures should obtain the annual returns published by the South African Nursing Council so that changes can be noted and trends observed. As more of the national states become independent and establish their own registering bodies the numbers reflected will undergo changes which must be viewed in the light of historic developments and not misinterpreted.

A decline in the number of persons registered or enrolled with the South African Nursing Council may not denote a real decrease in number of such persons, but merely that they no longer register in the Republic of South Africa but with their own registration body. The number making up the total population in the Republic will be affected as more national states gain independence.

Professional nurses in the Republic of South Africa occupy a wide variety of nursing posts. These include director of nursing services, deputy director of nursing services, chief nursing service manager, senior nursing service manager, nursing service manager, chief professional nurse, senior professional nurse, professor, senior lecturer, lecturer and junior lecturer. Other designations include district nurse, midwife and, in the sub-professional group, staff nurse. There are also special titles applicable to male nurses only. Nomenclature varies and undergoes changes to meet changing circumstances. Suffice it to say that professional nurses in the Republic of South Africa occupy positions of the greatest responsibility and are involved at the highest level in the policy-making bodies of almost all health care delivery systems.

The nursing profession in the Republic of South Africa is thus well supplied with persons who are well qualified to undertake the work required of them and who make a great contribution to the health care of all the diverse groups which make up the population of the Republic of South Africa. The social forces that shape the growth of the nursing profession will continue to exert an influence on the nursing profession in this country. It is a dynamic, ever-growing, ever-changing profession, composed of many people ready to accept change (and even to initiate it) and to take with them those who are not innovators, but, if ably led, render inestimable service for the benefit of those in need of health care, be it preventive, promotive, curative, maintenance or rehabilitative.

A PROFESSIONAL ASSOCIATION

Criterion 6, relating to the characteristics in terms of which a profession is appraised, stated that one such measure is 'self-organisation leading to the formation of a professional association and a self-governing body which controls professional standards'.

As has already been stated, the profession of nursing in South Africa measures up to both these requirements, the professional governing body being the South African Nursing Council which was established by Act 45 of 1944.

A professional association, the South African Trained Nurses' Association, was officially constituted on 1 October 1914. The aims of this association were:
- to weld the nurses of South Africa into one united bond of workers
- to encourage cooperation and to take united action for the protection of the profession
- to encourage and in every way maintain the highest ideals for nursing in South Africa
- to hold social and professional gatherings whenever necessary or expedient to discuss all matters pertaining to or affecting the interests of the profession
- to take such steps towards the formation of benevolent funds or pension schemes as may be thought necessary
- to become more actively united by means of similar nurses' organisations in other countries with the members of the profession throughout the world
- to take all possible steps to suppress the practice of nursing by unqualified women, and to prevent abuse of the nurse's uniform

and later also:
- to secure, promote and maintain legislative measures, or petition any government, legislative or administrative body to further the interests of nurses and midwives
- to provide a trained and qualified nursing service for the benefit and protection of the public.

These stated aims were fairly comprehensive and the Association did a great deal to put nursing on a proper professional footing in South Africa. It was due to its efforts that the Nursing Act was put forward and passed in 1944.

The South African Trained Nurses' Association was superseded by the South African Nursing Association, a statutory body constituted under Act 45 of 1944.

Rise of professional associations

The rise of professional associations started during the Middle Ages when the people who practised a particular craft or calling came together. Barristers and surgeons, formed like-interest associations fairly early, while members of church or university groups, such as physicians, did not feel the need for such bodies. It is part of history that when a new profession evolves within an existing one, it remains for some time within its parent profession and the establishment of the new one as a separate entity is retarded. This happened with dentistry as a branch of medicine, and with many others which today are regarded as specialist professions with their own associations. Colleges of specialities also grew up, for example the Royal College of Physicians. The aims of such colleges were to prevent malpractice and protect the public.

During the sixteenth century many of the old forms of association fell into disuse. A later development, during the eighteenth century, was the getting together of groups from the same field of work with the idea of creating a meeting place for friendly and convivial meetings. Dining clubs and the like were formed and social activities were paramount. As is natural, when people from the same walk of life meet frequently, informal although quite serious discussions arise regarding common problems. Study societies also became established. It was from such beginnings that professional associations owed their revival.

For the most part early associations or societies had a simple form of constitution and consisted of a single grade of members with perhaps some honorary members. These have evolved and continue to do so as society's needs and composition change.

Professional standards

The laying down of professional standards and testing of professional competence, which in many instances originally formed part of the associations' functions, became the work of other bodies, for the most part statutory bodies acting as another arm of the state. Thus in South Africa we have the South African Medical Council and the South African Nursing Council which control standards, inspect training schools and register practitioners, and the South African Medical Association and South African Nursing Association which are more concerned with the interests of practitioners of the profession and the advancement of the profession as such. At present special interest groups are catered for mainly by discussion groups acting through branches to headquarters of the South African Nursing Association.

Organisation of professional associations

The organisation and mode of functioning of professional associations, that is using the word association in its broadest sense as a linking together of persons to promote an objective or with common interest, of course varies, and evolves to meet change. An association may be of the federal or confederal type.

A federal association is a system of organisation in which a central overhead body or governing body has a number of different, smaller or even regional associations in membership. The constitution is so framed that the greatest possible measure of autonomy of action and decision-making is granted to the constituent associations. The powers, authority and duties of the central body and of the constituent associations are laid down in the constitutions of the central as well as the constituent member associations, and are guaranteed in the constitutions of each. A federation is a means of decentralisation or regionalisation without losing the overall unity necessary at national level.

A confederal association is a form of loosely bound associations which nevertheless have a common bond, aim or objective.

Nursing associations

Nursing associations throughout the world are undergoing reorganisation, for example the Canadian Nursing Association is now a confederation. The Royal College of Nursing (Rcn), in addition to its overhead central organisations, now has four major nursing associations under its aegis, namely those of nursing students, nursing management, nursing practice and nursing education. Each of these associations has local Rcn centres which are linked to regional committees and thus to the central body. Each has also developed special-interest societies within the membership structure.

Other examples that could be studied include the American Nurses' Association, which is composed of nurses' associations of the 50 states, each of which are again subdivided into district nurses' associations (which now number more than 800) and the National League for Nursing in America. The latter is a membership organisation of individuals and agencies. America also has other nurses' associations which are autonomous special-interest groups.

Whatever form professional associations take, they have the following characteristics in common:

- [ ] Stated aims or objectives
- [ ] A philosophy
- [ ] A constitution, regulations and rules of conduct of meetings, etc
- [ ] Members
- [ ] An organisational structure including a governing body
- [ ] Headquarters
- [ ] Activities related to their aims or objectives
- [ ] A means of financing their activities, such as membership dues, etc
- [ ] An official channel of communication with members, often in the form of a journal or newsletter
- [ ] Relationship with other organisations.

The functions of a professional nursing association include:

- [ ] the organisation of its members in order to enable them to carry out the stated objectives of the association
- [ ] the development of the profession through education and guidance of its members
- [ ] the promotion and preservation of the highest standards of professional conduct
- [ ] the raising of the status of the profession, including the socio-economic conditions of its members, and the undertaking of research into all matters related to nursing and nurses
- [ ] the protection of the profession against exploitation
- [ ] the preservation of the service motive and constant striving to improve the quality of service members can offer.

There are also international nursing organisations such as the International Council of Nurses, and the International Committee of Catholic Nurses.

Because disease, famine, ignorance and related health problems have existed throughout the world for many centuries, and because nurses have been vitally concerned with such matters, they have sought membership, either individually or through the affiliation of their own professional organisation, of other international groups concerned with health matters. These include the International Hospital Federation and the International Union for Health Education.

It will be seen that professional associations have many facets and can take on many forms.

The danger inherent in professional associations can be a built-in rigidity which makes it impossible for the association to remain in the mainstream of modern thought. This must be recognised and resisted if professional associations are to fulfil the needs for which they were created and truly meet one of the important criteria that comprise the hallmark of professionalism. In nursing the professional association continues to evolve in the same way as the dynamic profession itself does.

Professional associations develop a code of ethics by which nurses order their professional lives. Nurses in South Africa base their ethical code on the teachings of the religious sisterhoods which started professional nursing in South Africa, and on the precepts of the medical profession with which it has close links. Through a professional association, it must continue to strive for the best in professionalism.

5 Principles of professional practice in nursing

Some of the ideas expressed in this chapter originated out of lectures given by Professor C Searle which the author attended while studying for the MCur (Nursing Education) at the University of Pretoria. Ideas were also crystallised during discussions, seminars and assignments which were part of this study.

No book dealing with the profession of nursing would be complete without a chapter dealing specifically with the principles of professional practice in nursing, for this is the basis of the nurse's professional existence.

LEGAL ASPECTS

In all countries control of the practice of nursing is aimed at the protection of the public and any legislation is directed towards this goal. Many countries have passed legislation dealing with nurses' practice. These acts vary considerably in content and application. Most make provision for registration of practitioners of nursing with a controlling body. This book is concerned with the South African nursing field only and therefore no further mention of other countries will be made here. (For details of the historical aspects relating to South Africa, see Searle 1965.)

South Africa was the first country in the world to obtain state registration for nurses in 1891. She was followed by Britain, various states in America, and Canada. Other countries became aware of the necessity for control of nursing practice and registration of properly qualified nurses and enacted their own legislation. The first South African legislation providing for state registration of nurses and midwives was incorporated in the *Medical and Pharmacy Act,* 1891 (Act 34 of 1891) of the Cape Colony, and the registering body was the Colonial Medical Council. The nurses of the Republics and what was then Rhodesia made use of this registration facility, but by the time nursing in that province had developed so far as to require recognition of training, Natal already had its own medical council.

The registration of nurses and midwives by legislation accorded recognition of professional status to nurses. Regulations were made under the Act, which provided for the mechanism of registration, the nature of the course of training, examination systems, an ethical code and disciplinary control. At first registration was voluntary. This meant that persons who met the registration requirements in respect of training and education and testing for competence could apply for registration. Many already trained nurses did so, but others did not. There is thus a clear distinction between a trained nurse and a registered nurse. A registered nurse must meet laid down training requirements so that a registered nurse is always trained, but a trained nurse need not always be a registered nurse. Anyone not registered with the controlling body is not entitled to use the term *registered nurse*.

In 1910 the four colonies of South Africa were united into the Union of South Africa, but it was not until the enactment of the *Medical, Dental and Pharmacy Act*, 1928 (Act 13 of 1928) that a consolidating law replaced the separate provincial registrations. The South African Medical Council became the controlling and registering body, with powers of registration, approval of training, examination, certificate granting and disciplinary control. This Act included a very important provision, namely the 'prescribing' of certain areas by proclamation so that only persons registered under the Act in a specific category of nursing might practise nursing for gain in that area. This paved the way for subsequent developments, the first of which was the enactment of the *Nursing Act*, 1944 (Act 69 of 1944), which placed the control of the nursing profession in the hands of nurses and made the South African Nursing Council the registering and disciplinary body, with its own examining powers or recognition of the examinations of other bodies.

The Nursing Act was amended several times, re-enacted as Act 69 of 1957 and amended again, particularly significantly by the *Nursing Amendment Act*, 1972 (Act 50 of 1972), which finally made it illegal for anyone to practise nursing for gain unless registered or enrolled with the South African Nursing Council. This includes all categories of nurses and midwives from the professional registered nurse, through the enrolled nurse to the enrolled nursing assistant. Students and pupils also have to be registered or enrolled with the South African Nursing Council. The provisions of the Act are enforced by the courts of law.

The Nursing Act in force is Act 50 of 1978 as amended by the *Nursing Amendment Act*, 1981 (Act 71 of 1981). It is the professional responsibility of every practitioner to keep up to date with amendments and changes in the Act as these occur. It is fundamental to professional practice that nurses are thoroughly conversant with the legal requirements concerning the practice of their profession and that they abide by these legal requirements, which include the regulations made under the Act. The following provision is of particular importance.

☐ *Maintenance of registration or enrolment* The nurse has a personal responsibility to see to it that she is legally entitled to practise by maintaining her registration or enrolment. This is her professional duty, fundamental to professional practice, and is not the responsibility of the employing body whose only task is to see to it that persons who are not legally empowered to practise because of failure to ensure that their registration or enrolment is duly maintained, are not employed.

Professional misconduct is dealt with by the disciplinary powers vested in the controlling body. A nurse is also a citizen and is subject to the same laws as other citizens. Besides criminal proceedings, the nurse guilty of an offence may have to face disciplinary action by her own controlling body.

After a duly constituted disciplinary inquiry, if found guilty of improper or disgraceful conduct the nurse may be punished in various ways.

A nurse may not practise as a doctor. However, she works *with* a doctor and not *under* him. She remains personally responsible for the manner in which she carries out her duties and for recording her actions. She may take a prescription from a doctor for the treatment of *his* patient, who is also *her* patient. When an act is illegal she may not take a prescription or order it. When a nurse does not know how to carry out an act she should not accept the prescription for treatment, but should tell the doctor that she does not know how to do it.

Her independent functions, that is those that do not require a prescription or order from a doctor or dentist, are her own responsibility, with the proviso that the patient is the doctor's patient as well as her patient and her actions form part of the therapeutic programme as a whole. These must complement those of the doctor.

THE INDEPENDENT, INTERDEPENDENT AND DEPENDENT FUNCTIONS OF A NURSE

In 1982 *Professor Charlotte Searle*, with her usual insight, clarified thought on these functions of the nurse. In the past it was customary to talk of the independent and dependent functions of the nurse without examining the subject in depth. Today health care is given in a team context. Each member has a specific role and function, with a legal right to practise. The medical practitioner has specific levels of expertise that lead him to make the major diagnostic and therapeutic decisions, decisions that will be implemented largely by other members of the health team who are then accountable for their own actions. One of these persons is the nurse, whose functions will now be examined.

The independent functions of a nurse

These may be listed as follows:

☐ *Supervision of the patient or client so as to ensure his safety and security* This includes aspects such as asepsis and cleanliness, which are part of the safe environment, and security from physical as well as emotional hazards. The patient must be unable to injure himself or others. Safety includes ensuring that the patient is clearly identified.

☐ *Observation of patient or client* This includes signs and symptoms of disease, any change in the patient's condition during the course of the illness or treatment, and any reactions, untoward or otherwise that may occur.

☐ *Recording and reporting* Observations made, instructions received and given, care and treatment carried out (including the patient's reactions to treatment or other events) must be recorded and reported accurately, precisely and in such a manner that they are easily understood by those who have to read them and carry on with treatment.

- *Assessment of the patient's response to treatment* Decisions that will involve changes in the planned therapeutic programme may have to be taken as a result of this assessment.
- *Nursing diagnosis* This may be for nursing care, for referral to a medical practitioner, or for emergency action by the nurse before a medical practitioner arrives on the scene.
- *Performing nursing procedures* The nurse must perform the nursing procedures required by the treatment prescribed, the condition of the patient or client, the reason underlying the procedure, the availability of equipment and other factors. Nursing procedures must be carried out accurately, with competence and with due regard for the patient's physical and mental comfort and his safety. Record-keeping is also necessary.
- *Supervision of personnel* This is necessary so that duties are delegated to persons with the knowledge and ability to carry them out. Teaching staff members is an important part of supervision.
- *Education of the patient/client and his relatives or friends* This is to ensure that, where possible, self-care is undertaken, that therapy is continued for as long as is necessary and that community resources are known to the person being treated or to those caring for him in the home and are used when and as the need arises. Preventive aspects of health care must be emphasised.

Thus eight independent functions of the nurse have been identified. Many interrelate as interaction takes place between other members of the health team. The nurse does not need a prescription to know that she must observe the patient's condition carefully after surgery. It is part of her independent professional responsibility to do so.

The interdependent functions of a nurse

These relate to the interrelationships between the nurse and the patient and the nurse and other members of the health team, particularly the interdependence of nursing and medicine. Neither the nurse nor the doctor can provide all the health care that the patient needs. Coordination of activities and acknowledgement of each other's field of expertise is essential.

In modern practice, with its comprehensive approach, this is one of the most important functions.

The dependent functions of a nurse

The dependent functions of a nurse are based on the law that authorises her practice as well as on common law and relevant statutory laws. The Nursing Act, as amended from time to time, is the law that empowers the nurse to practise, and the regulations promulgated in terms of the Act govern this practice. It is the law, and *only the law*, that authorises the professional practice of the nurse.

There are other Acts that have to be taken into consideration, such as those governing the control and handling of medicines, and it is the nurse's duty to be aware of her responsibilities under common law and laws specifically affecting health care. Ultimately the nurse, practising within legal boundaries, is responsible for her own acts. Whether she practices within an institution or as a private contractor, she remains personally responsible and accountable to the registration authority which, in South Africa, is the South African Nursing Council. She is also answerable, in the broader sense, to the courts of law.

The nurse herself is the only one who can be held personally responsible for her actions. Inefficient work on her part becomes the concern of the doctor and the employing authority if reported. She is accountable for the type of care she gives in carrying out a prescription. Her acceptance of a doctor's prescription for patient care constitutes an unwritten agreement between professional colleagues. She accepts the order and must see that it is carried out. No other person, be he or she senior to the nurse in question, may interfere with the order and attempt to change it.

The legislation that gives nurses the legal right to practise nursing for gain, subject to certain stipulations, means that nurses can carry out nursing practice for the benefit of the community. Nursing is a service indispensable to mankind and as such has ethical standards of professional practice that have evolved over time and must be part of the philosophy and the lifestyle of every professional nurse. (Ethical aspects are discussed in more detail in chapter 6.)

The original Nursing Act brought into being two statutory bodies, namely:

☐ the South African Nursing Council (SANC)
☐ the South African Nursing Association (SANA).

THE SOUTH AFRICAN NURSING COUNCIL (SANC)

The prime concern of this body is the welfare of the public served by nurses. It lays down minimum periods of education and training for licensing of the various categories of nurses, ensures the maintenance of ethical standards and registers or enrols nurses, depending on their education and training. Thus the public is guaranteed that registered nurses, enrolled nurses and enrolled nursing assistants are adequately prepared by prescribed, approved programmes and that upon satisfactory completion of these programmes they have been registered or enrolled. Once registered or enrolled, nurses have to maintain this registration by paying an annual fee.

The SANC lays down the *scope of practice* of the various categories of nurse. It is important that students preparing for registration and pupils preparing for enrolment are made aware of these provisions before they go into practice.

The SANC, as stated earlier, also exercises a *disciplinary function*. After being charged and given a hearing before a disciplinary committee of her peers, if *found guilty* a nurse may:
- be cautioned *or* reprimanded
- be cautioned *and* reprimanded
- be *suspended for a specific period of time* from practising as a nurse
- have her name *removed* from the register or roll (this excludes any practice until such time as the Council, on application, sees fit to restore her name to the register or a roll, which requires full Council approval
- in the case of a student or pupil, have the period of education and training extended.

Composition of the SANC

The South African Nursing Council consists of 30 members, 20 of whom are appointed by various bodies or persons. Ten registered nurses are elected by the profession from among its members. Of the 20 appointed members, seven must be registered nurses and six may be medical practitioners *or* registered nurses. This means that the composition of 30 members includes at least 17 registered nurses, with the possibility of a further 8 (6 + 2) optional appointments. Thus the Council *must* have 17 registered nurse members and *may* have 25 registered nurse members. The Council is multiracial.

The Council elects from among its members a president and a vice-president (who must be nurses) and a treasurer. In addition it appoints a registrar, who is a full-time paid official responsible for the administrative functions of the Council. He is assisted by a staff of full-time, paid officials and others necessary to the efficient carrying out of the Council's activities.

Activities of the SANC

- *Maintaining the registers and rolls* of duly qualified members. These include the:
    - Register of nurses
    - Register of student nurses
    - Roll of enrolled nurses
    - Roll of pupil enrolled nurses
    - Roll of nursing assistants
    - Roll of pupil nursing assistants

as well as the registers of midwives, psychiatric nurses, community nurses and registered nurses (General, Psychiatric, Community) and midwives from the new comprehensive course.

There are also registers for those holding additional qualifications, such as tutors and nurse administrators, as well as qualifications in clinical fields such as intensive nursing, orthopaedic nursing, ophthalmic nursing, paediatric nursing, clinical care, administration and instruction, operating theatre nursing, advanced midwifery and neonatal nursing, advanced psychiatric nursing, oncology nursing, advanced paediatric and neonatal nursing, clinical nursing, health assessment, treatment and care, geriatric nursing, renal nursing, etc.

- ☐ *Collecting fees* All registered and enrolled nurses *must maintain registration or enrolment* by paying an annual fee to the SANC in order to be legally entitled to practise their profession. (Students and pupils pay a fee at the commencement of a course and then on registration or enrolment, after which they are liable to annual payment like all other registered or enrolled nurses.)
- ☐ *Removing names from registers or rolls* The SANC can remove names from the registers or rolls for the following reasons:
  - Failure to pay the fee by the due date.
  - On request of a nurse, for example when she marries and stops practising as a nurse, because of ill-health, retirement, etc.
  - As a result of disciplinary action.
  - Failure to notify change of address which leads to failure to pay annual fees.

A nurse is guilty of a criminal offence if she practises nursing for gain (in cash or kind) or holds herself out to be a registered or enrolled nurse when she is *not*, in fact, on the register or roll of the SANC, as the case may be.

- ☐ Appointing examiners and moderators where Council conducts examinations, conducting examinations and granting of diplomas or certificates.
- ☐ Establishing disciplinary committees to deal with alleged misconduct.
- ☐ Establishing an education committee.
- ☐ Approving nursing schools and inspecting such schools (the SANC has recently expanded its professional department to make inspection functions as well as assistance to training schools and not just examination functions a reality), approving education and training programmes, inspecting institutions offering programmes of education and training of any category of nurse, including post-registration qualifications.
- ☐ Issuing or renewing licences to carry on the business of a nursing agency and inspecting the running of such agencies.
- ☐ Considering any matters affecting the nursing or midwifery professions and making representations or taking any action in connection with those that, as a Council, it may deem advisable.
- ☐ Making regulations in order to carry out its functions (important ones are those concerning the election procedure, procedure for disciplinary committee meetings, regulations for the practice of midwifery, regulations regarding the wearing of distinguishing devices and uniforms for various categories of nurses, regulations relating to the keeping, supply, administering or prescribing of medicines by registered nurses, rules setting out the acts or omissions in respect of which the Council may take disciplinary steps, regulations for the education and training of various

categories of nurses, regulations relating to the scope of practice of persons who are registered or enrolled under the Act and others).

Three of these regulations will be discussed in some detail as they are of vital importance to those studying to become practitioners of nursing, registered or enrolled.

I Rules regarding acts and omissions in respect of which the council may take disciplinary steps (R387 – 15 Feb 1985 as amended by R866 of 24 April 1987)

At the moment this regulation, in Chapter 2, deals only with the acts and omissions in respect of which the Council may take disciplinary steps against a *registered nurse*. The student should have a copy of these and study them thoroughly, as they are vital to her future practice.

II Scope of practice of persons who are registered or enrolled under the Nursing Act, 1978 (R2598 – 30 Nov 1984 as amended by R1469 of 10 July 1987)

These regulations set out in detail, for the first time in South Africa, the scope of practice of registered nurses and registered midwives.

For discussion of the scope of practice of registered nurses see Searle, *Professional Practice* chapter 13.

All those preparing for registration should obtain the regulations relating to the scope of practice of registered nurses, and enrolled categories when these are promulgated, and study them carefully. A registered person *must* obtain these regulations and *must* keep herself up to date with any changes that occur in the future. It is the duty of registered (and enrolled) nurses to be aware of their duties and of any limitations with regard to the laid-down scope of practice.

The South African Nursing Council Professional Division

In March 1983 the SA Nursing Council decided to re-introduce a professional division within the personnel structure of the council. The functions of this division are:

☐ inspection and guidance to nursing schools

☐ assistance with the examination system of the Council (with the exception of the administrative section)

☐ professional assistance to the education committee

☐ attendance at meetings as instructed

☐ evaluation of overseas qualifications

☐ any other professional duties as instructed.

The division now consists of a chief professional officer and four others, each with specific responsibilities.

THE SOUTH AFRICAN NURSING ASSOCIATION[1]

The first *Nursing Act* (Act 45 of 1944) established both the South African Nursing Council and the South African Nursing Association.

The South African Nursing Association (SANA) is the national professional association which superseded the South African Trained Nurses Association (SATNA) in 1944. It acts as the official mouthpiece of the nursing profession and protects and promotes the interests of all nurses.

The SANA, as defined in Section 38 of the *Nursing Act* (Act 50 of 1978) as amended, represents the professions of nursing and midwifery in the Republic of South Africa. According to the Act membership is compulsory for all persons registered or enrolled under the Act and practising the profession for gain within the Republic.

The objectives of the Association are:
- to assist with the development of an adequate, efficient and effective nursing service for the Republic of South Africa
- to raise the status, maintain the integrity and promote the interests of the profession of nursing and midwifery
- to consider and deal with any matter concerning or affecting the profession of nursing and midwifery
- to perform acts necessary or incidental to the attainment of the above objects and to safeguard and further the interests of the Association and its members.

SANA negotiates on matters of general concern to the profession such as conditions of service, education and the nurse's role within the health team. In order to do this SANA negotiates with authorities such as the Department of National Health and Population Development and other government departments (when necessary and appropriate), private organisations, universities and the South African Nursing Council. Such negotiations are backed by extensive investigation, supported by numerous memoranda and involve lengthy discussion. Some matters that have been dealt with over the years include parity of salaries for nurses of different population groups, now largely achieved; improved salary scales, an ongoing activity; better leave facilities; pensions and hours of duty; and many more.

Improved education and training facilities for all categories of nurses, including post-registration specialisation courses, and degree study have all received attention over the years. Many changes and improvements have been brought about to date.

SANA also runs an advisory service, a professional indemnity scheme, a group personal benefit scheme and a Nurses' Trust Fund which cares for aged and disabled members. It has its own newspaper, the *Nursing News*, runs a specialised research library, the CA Nothard Library, administers numerous scholarships and bursaries, and runs a publication section, publishing local nursing literature and stocking other local and imported publications on nursing and related health matters.

It is clear that SANA is concerned chiefly with the welfare of nurses as a whole, for a well cared-for profession can provide effective and efficient care, while SANC has as its primary concern the welfare and protection of the public at large.

1 Information mainly from the South African Nursing Association 1986. 'A guide for Members'.

Organisation of the South African Nursing Association

In 1982 the South African Nursing Association began to function under a new Constitution. This Constitution provides for decentralisation to achieve greater involvement and communication and for direct representation of all population groups on regional boards and the Central Board.

Structure of the South African Nursing Association

Figure 5.1 Policy-making body (elected)

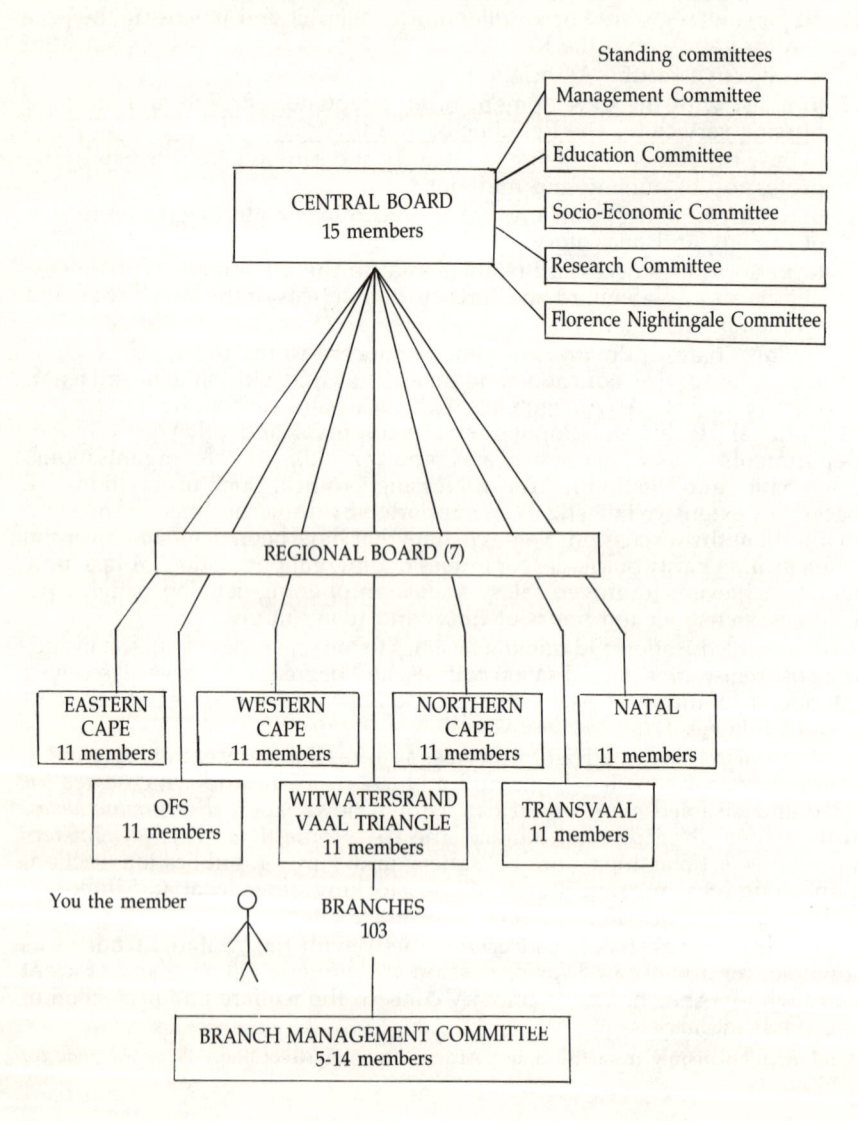

```
                                          Standing committees
                                          ┌─────────────────────────────┐
                                          │ Management Committee        │
                                          ├─────────────────────────────┤
                                          │ Education Committee         │
        ┌──────────────────┐              ├─────────────────────────────┤
        │  CENTRAL BOARD   │──────────────│ Socio-Economic Committee    │
        │    15 members    │              ├─────────────────────────────┤
        └──────────────────┘              │ Research Committee          │
                                          ├─────────────────────────────┤
                                          │ Florence Nightingale Committee │
                                          └─────────────────────────────┘

        ┌──────────────────────────────────────────┐
        │           REGIONAL BOARD (7)             │
        └──────────────────────────────────────────┘

  ┌──────────┐  ┌──────────┐  ┌──────────┐  ┌──────────┐
  │ EASTERN  │  │ WESTERN  │  │ NORTHERN │  │  NATAL   │
  │  CAPE    │  │  CAPE    │  │  CAPE    │  │          │
  │11 members│  │11 members│  │11 members│  │11 members│
  └──────────┘  └──────────┘  └──────────┘  └──────────┘

       ┌──────────┐  ┌──────────────┐  ┌──────────┐
       │   OFS    │  │ WITWATERSRAND│  │TRANSVAAL │
       │          │  │ VAAL TRIANGLE│  │          │
       │11 members│  │  11 members  │  │11 members│
       └──────────┘  └──────────────┘  └──────────┘

  You the member        BRANCHES
                          103

                ┌─────────────────────────────────┐
                │ BRANCH MANAGEMENT COMMITTEE     │
                │         5-14 members            │
                └─────────────────────────────────┘
```

Branches

It can be seen from figure 5.1 that the whole structure of the organisation rests on its branches, of which there are approximately 103 throughout the country at present. Each member is assigned to a branch in her geographical area.

Branches meet monthly or bi-monthly and it is at this level that the individual nurse is involved in the affairs of her Association and profession. Branch matters are managed by a branch management committee which is elected annually. The committee consists of not more than 11 and not less than five registered nurses, a student nurse, an enrolled nurse and an enrolled nursing assistant. The committee elects registered nurses from amongst its members to serve as chairman and vice-chairman.

Branches are consulted on various matters by regional boards and the Central Board. Branches may also refer matters to their regional board, and biennial regional meetings are held to which branches send delegates.

Regional boards

The overall control of the affairs of the Association in the seven regions is vested in the regional boards, subject to certain directions from the Central Board. A regional board must refer any matter that affects the profession as a whole to the Central Board.

A regional board consists of 11 members, nominated and elected by registered nurses of the region, who are paid-up members of the Association. Provision is made for representation of the different population groups as well as of nurses working in the public, private and educational sectors. In the event of 11 members not being nominated and elected, the regional board may, in consultation with the Central Board, appoint members.

The term of office of a regional board is four years and it meets at least twice a year. At the first meeting a regional board elects a chairman, vice-chairman and treasurer.

Central Board

The overall control of the Association is vested in the Central Board. It consists of 15 members of whom seven are the chairmen of the regional boards. The other eight members are elected by and from amongst the members of the regional boards.

The term of office of the Central Board is four years and it meets at least twice a year. At the first meeting of a new Board the President, Vice-President and Treasurer of the Association are elected by secret ballot.

The Central Board must consult with branches, via regional boards, on important policy matters. Such matters include amendment of the Association's Constitution, amendments to Acts that affect the nursing profession, increases in membership fees, non-administrative matters with far-reaching financial implications and policy statements of the South African Nursing Association.

The object of regionalisation was to bring the affairs of the Association closer to the members by giving them easier access to managers and other personnel in regional offices and taking away the feeling that the Association was some 'remote body' situated in Pretoria.

There are seven regional offices administered by regional managers and they are situated in Cape Town (Goodwood), Port Elizabeth, Kimberley, Bloemfontein, Durban, Johannesburg and Pretoria.

The main functions of the regional managers are:
- [ ] execution of the Association's business in the region
- [ ] liaison with members in the region
- [ ] to offer assistance to members in the region who have professional problems
- [ ] to identify expectations and needs in the region.

Head Office

The Head Office of the Association is situated in Pretoria. The chief executive officer is the Executive Director who is a registered nurse. The activities are divided into five main sections.

- [ ] *General administrative section* Activities under this section include:
  - member administration
  - personnel administration
  - financial administration
  - annual budget.
- [ ] *Training and development section* Functions under this section include:
  - determination of educational and developmental needs
  - professional training and development of members
  - library
  - publications department
  - administration of bursaries.
- [ ] *Socio-economic section* Functions in this section include:
  - improvement of the position of nurses
  - negotiations regarding conditions of service, salaries, benefits, indemnity issues, support services, etc.
- [ ] *Research section* Functions under this section include:
  - compilation of a National Nursing Research Register
  - specific research projects
  - promoting and utilising research and research results.
- [ ] *Communications department* Activities under this section include:
  - liaison with the public and organisations outside the profession
  - liaison with members and organisations within the profession
  - production and distribution of publications and information
  - enhancing the image of the nursing profession.

The Central Board appoints five standing committees:

- *The Management Committee* This is a small committee consisting of the three office bearers of the Central Board. A maximum of two additional members of the Central Board may be co-opted. The management committee attends to urgent matters which arise from time to time and cannot be dealt with by the executive staff. It may not take decisions regarding important policy matters, and all its decisions must be confirmed by the Central Board.
- *The Education Committee* This Committee is a working committee established for the purpose of assisting the Central Board to achieve its objects in respect of progress in the field of education regarding an adequate, efficient and effective nursing service for South Africa which keeps abreast of developments in the health services.
- *The Socio-economic Committee* This Committee deals with matters of social and economic concern to nurses such as salaries and conditions of service.
- *The Research Committee* This Committee is a working committee established for the purpose of assisting the Central Board to achieve its objectives in respect of developing nursing research.
- *The Florence Nightingale Committee* The awarding of most of the bursaries administered by the Association is undertaken by this Committee.

Administrative structure

The Central Board and regional boards maintain offices and appoint full-time staff to carry out their decisions and to administer the affairs of the Association. All services to members are available in both official languages.

OTHER POINTS OF IMPORTANCE IN PROFESSIONAL PRACTICE

The following aspects which come into the practice of the profession of nursing are of particular concern to all practitioners:
- *Maintenance of professional competence* Every nurse who continues to practise her profession has a moral obligation to keep herself up to date with developments in her chosen field by reading, discussion, inquiry and attendance at seminars, symposia or short courses that are available from time to time. In fact, if opportunities are not there the professional nurse should create them.
- *Maintenance and control of practice* so that the highest standard of care is available to clients and patients at all times. This entails supervision of personnel working under the direction of professionals and the allocation of duties in a responsible manner.
- *Maintenance at all times* of measures that will ensure the safety of the patient or client's person, name and property. This includes not only *wilful* injury or loss or damage to possessions, but also *negligence* which leads to harm to the patient's person, name, or property. Neglect can be established only if the person *performing* the act had a duty to take care and there was an absence of such care which caused actual damage as a direct result of absence of such care.

Figure 5.2 Administrative structure of the South African Nursing Association

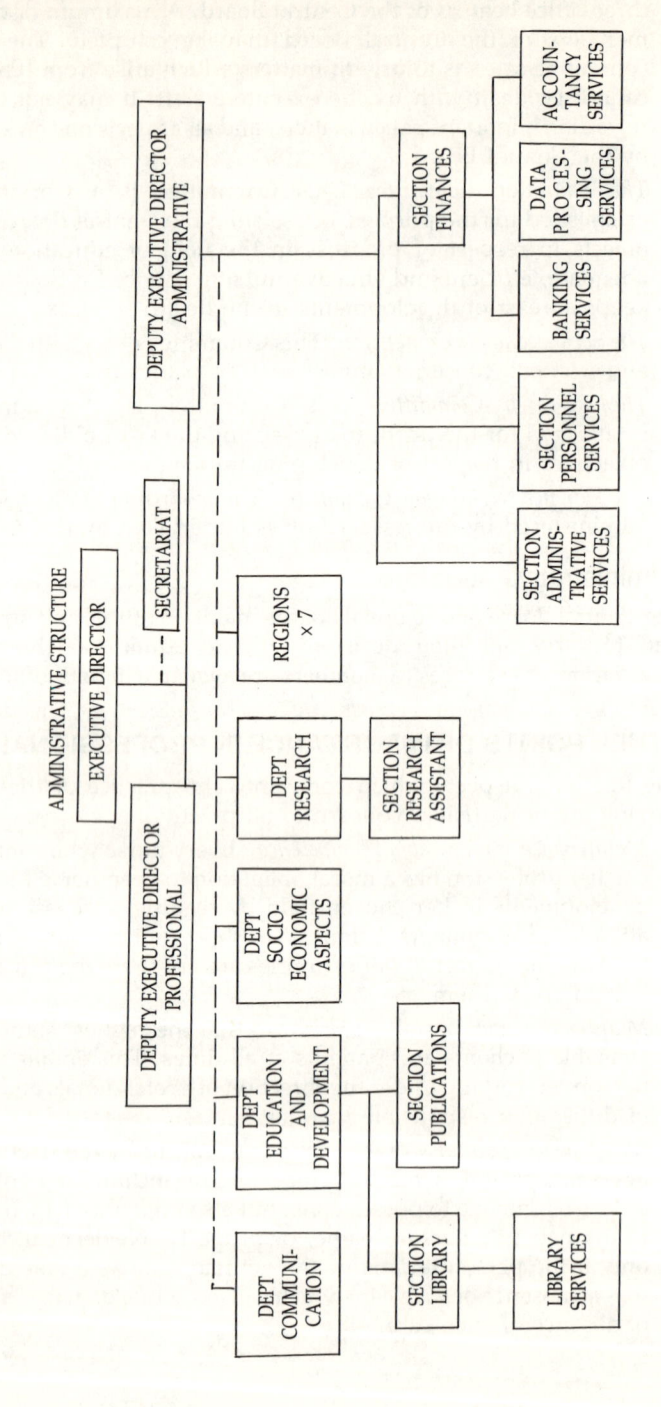

- *Fulfilment of contractual obligations* A contract is (according to Searle) an agreement between two or more persons whereby one or more of them promises to give something to or to do something for the other. Thus a nurse applying for a post who is appointed and accepts the post with a due date for assuming duty has entered into a contract.
- *Ensuring that continuous service is maintained* when a patient needs it. Thus a professional nurse does not walk off duty if her relief has not arrived and the patient needs service. Adequate relief must be obtained first.
- *Carrying out medical prescriptions, requests or directions* with intelligence and integrity. This includes observation, reporting and record-keeping.
- *Maintenance of confidence* in the doctor and other members of the health team.
- *Avoidance* of the use of their names or pictures in connection with advertisements.
- *Acceptance only of the type of compensation* for her services that is implied in the contract. Tips, bribes, etc cannot be taken.
- *Provision of a full day's work for a full day's pay* The need to fulfil her part of the bargain with her employing body or person is a basic requirement.
- *Maintenance of standards of behaviour* which are accepted norms in the community.
- *Non-participation in public political activities and demonstrations* A patient must never feel threatened by a nurse displaying obvious partiality.
- *Maintenance of a high standard of role image* by the nurse at all times.
- *Intelligent acceptance of legitimate authority and discipline* This does not imply slavish obedience, but adherence to rules and regulations for the common good, always with the proviso that considered judgment must be exercised.
- *Maintenance of good interpersonal relationships* between clients, patients and all members of the health care team.
- *Taking the necessary measures* to ensure that the practitioner's health is maintained at an optimal level and ensuring, if deviation from health occurs, that it in no way endangers the safety of those committed to her care or that of her colleagues in the health care delivery team.
- *Maintenance at all times of the utmost respect* for the basic human worth and dignity of all committed to the care of the professional nurse.
- *Practice of economy* within the bounds of safe practice.
- *Education of neophytes* in the profession.

All these and many more go to up make the practice of the profession of nursing.

It is hoped that this section has given the student an insight into the two bodies that are of concern to her professional practice, and into professional practice in nursing in general.

6 The ethical basis of the profession of nursing

The major revision of this chapter is largely the work of Mrs Una Brown, senior lecturer in the Department of Nursing, University of Cape Town.

Ethics is a word frequently bandied about without any real appreciation of its meaning. A little time spent on the clarification of this concept should be of value before going further into the ethical basis of the nursing profession.

Ethics is a moral philosophy, the philosophy of behaviour or conduct. It formulates principles upon which man bases his actions.

The word 'ethic' is derived from the Greek *ethikos*, meaning custom or character, and is defined as the science of morals. It is more commonly used in the form 'ethics', which is defined as the science of human conduct and character. It does not consider human conduct and character *per se*, but considers these two concepts in the light of moral judgements which have been passed upon them from time to time. It is a universal and practical science which deals with elements common to the entire human race.

THE ORIGIN OF ETHICS AS A SCIENCE

This goes back as far as the time when man was first able to ask 'Why?' When confronted with alternative ways of responding to a situation he must have tried out each until he found what seemed to him the best way of carrying out an action. This is relatively easy when deciding which is the right or wrong way of moving a stone, but when human relationships are involved the right and wrong way of acting, behaving or living is not so easy to determine.

The concept of right and wrong in human conduct, which is the field of study of ethics, has been influenced by facts, fashions, customs and traditional codes of conduct built up through the ages, from prescientific times to today. It constantly undergoes revision.

Basically there are three kinds of judgement applied to human conduct. There are acts that:

- ☐ a human being *should* perform
- ☐ a human being should *not* perform
- ☐ allow the human being a *choice* of either performing or not performing them.

If only it was as simple and clear-cut as that – Black and white, wrong and right! In life there are so many grey areas, so many factors that cloud the issue.

When considering nursing ethics this must be recognised. There will be some actions that will *universally* be regarded as *right*, and others that will *universally* be regarded as *wrong*. However, when the actions of the professional person, who is also a human being with human failings and frailties, are judged, it is those actions performed consciously and wilfully, and for which the performer can be held accountable, that are taken into account. Very brief consideration will make it abundantly clear that there are many areas in medical and nursing practice that are likely to present problems in the work situation.

Legal aspects also come into consideration, but civil law requirements and moral judgement do not always coincide. Obviously there are legal restrictions that will affect nursing practice and will be rigorously adhered to, but there are many areas in modern medical practice that give rise to conflicts. Medical power has become so great – keeping people alive on machines, treating conditions which only a few decades ago were untreatable – that questions such as 'Must I because I can?' are posed with ever-increasing frequency.

To return to the consideration of the study of ethics itself, let us regard it as *'the practical study of the norms and values which guide the judgement of what is right and what is wrong in human conduct'*.

The added question of whether this conduct is reasonable or can reasonably be expected from a human being also comes into play. In general the study of ethics falls into three categories, namely descriptive, normative and analytical ethics (meta-ethics).

Descriptive ethics

This embodies what the name implies, that is it is concerned with a description of the values and beliefs of various cultural, religious or social groups regarding the meaning of disease and the attitude of the group towards suffering, the group norms in respect of the care of the terminally ill and the values and norms governing the care of the aged.

If we study the findings of persons concerned with descriptive ethics this knowledge can help us to understand the expectations of people who come to us for care. Nurses have to deal with people from different cultures and different social backgrounds. These people interpret illness and health differently according to the value and norms of their own groups and cultures. Their attitudes, which are internalised, may make their reaction to illness, safety measures, health precautions and other matters affecting health care, differ widely. The knowledge of how various ethnic or religious groups feel they should act or of what is right for them enables health care professionals to understand and therefore to provide improved care for patients and clients.

Normative ethics

This is a study of human activities in a broad sense in an attempt to determine what constitutes right or wrong human actions and good or bad human qualities. It attempts to establish what is right and wrong for the human beings with whom we come into contact. Health in our modern Western culture is regarded as the *right* of all and ill-health as a *wrong*.

This is not true of all cultures, nor has it always been so of Western cultures. Before medical knowledge was so advanced health was regarded as *good fortune* and not something that could be acquired and maintained. To a certain extent this attitude is still evident today, for example the view that 'He is lucky to be so well!'

Normative ethics also includes the consideration of the legal implications of practice. When applied to nursing, normative ethics addresses issues such as:

☐ What should be the scope of practice of the various categories of nurses after having undertaken different nursing courses?

☐ What levels of competence can be expected of each of these categories?

☐ When can a nurse legally be regarded as having been negligent?

This leads to the concept of professional accountability, which will be discussed in another chapter.

Analytical ethics

Analytical ethics seeks to analyse the meanings of moral terms. It attempts not only to determine what is right and wrong, but also to seek justification for why these are correct or incorrect actions or attitudes. Nursing, indeed any form of health care is a *service* to people in *need* of that care, the *service* motive being paramount.

Nurses render a service of a particular and unique kind. This is their whole *raison d'être*. That they are recompensed for their service or benefit from it is of secondary importance. This does not mean that nurses should not be adequately rewarded for their services, but such reward should not be the overriding motive for them providing that service if they would call themselves professionals.

PROFESSIONAL ETHICS

In the practice of her profession the nurse must be guided by a *code of professional ethics*. 'Professional ethics is a type of applied normative ethics which applies ethical principles and rules that determine which actions are right and which are wrong to particular problem areas' (Smith *et al* 1985:336). Nursing ethics falls into this category.

Nursing ethics

Nursing ethics must not be confused with nursing etiquette, which is the unwritten code of professional conduct. Nursing etiquette is a local and private matter, concerned with courtesy to fellow workers.

Nursing ethics, on the other hand, is not a private concern, either of the individual practitioner or of the profession. 'Professional ethics develops in dialogue with society and is open to public scrutiny' (Jameton, A (1984), quoted in Smith *et al* 1985: 336). By this it is meant that nurses are expected by their peers to have been successfully socialised into the profession and to have internalised norms and values which are then reflected in the manner in which they conduct themselves in professional situations. However, because we are all individuals each nurse will perforce choose to do this in a different, unique, individual and creative way. This should be encouraged, but with the proviso that her behaviour remains within the limitations determined by her peers and her profession.

The South African ethical codes of nursing practice are currently being challenged by rapid and drastic socio-politico-economic changes in society. Because a tacit social contract between society and the nursing profession is implied and necessary if a nurse is to meet the health needs of the community successfully, the implications of these social changes must be reflected in current ethical codes of nursing practice. This has made it imperative for nurses in South Africa to evaluate the existing codes, recommend their updating and encourage the debating of ethical issues by nurses.

> Nursing ethics has the particular responsibility within nursing to examine critically the ethical dimensions of nursing practice with regard to its theories, diagnostic categories, diagnostic procedures, treatment goals and treatment procedures. In order to accomplish these tasks nurses must become more knowledgeable in the ethical analysis of nursing practice. Nurse ethicists must emerge to assist in this endeavour. And finally, nursing must forge strong inter-disciplinary ties to develop opportunities for dialogue about these concerns in other disciplines and various sectors of society (Smith *et al* 1985: 339).

Ethics is based on principles and principles do not change because the work site changes. The same principles apply whether the nurse works in a hospital or in a community.

Codes of nursing ethics

Various attempts have been made to codify these principles. 'Codes do not remain static but evolve with society and with the profession's role in society' (Smith *et al*: 336). The evolution of nursing ethical codes will be evident from a comparison of the various codes of ethics (see Appendix D).

Medical ethics

'Medical ethics, bound within the moral principles of the society in which medicine is being practised, has evolved slowly over the centuries from the Code of Hammurabi in 2000 BCE through the Ten Commandments in 1500 BCE, the Hippocratic Code (460-377 BCE) to several more recent declarations such as the WHO Declaration of Geneva in 1948, the Declaration of Helsinki and the Nuremburg Code which express heightened responsiveness to the needs and rights of patients as individuals' (Benatar 1986: 5).

Nurses should have knowledge of the evolution of medical codes of practice and of the concerns facing medical ethicists if they are to forge strong interdisciplinary ties so as to develop opportunities for dialogue which may be helpful in the ethical analysis of nursing practice.

Demographic transition, an aspect of social change, with its concomitant problems such as the unprecedented population increase which started round about the eighteenth century, urbanisation, poor sanitation, overcrowding, disease, technological development and the industrial revolution has, over the years, presented the medical profession with specific professional responsibilities and with ethical and legal problems (Baly 1986: 20). As the practice of medicine has changed to accommodate the changing needs of society, it has gained increasing medical power. It is this power which presents the profession with moral dilemmas.

'Moral dilemmas in medicine arise when there are two alternative choices about right and wrong actions, neither of which seems completely satisfactory. The choices involve putting one set of values up against another' (Benatar 1986: 7). In such instances moral codes such as the Hippocratic Oath are too limited for modern medical practice, but do still provide guidelines for moral decisions and modern codes of medical ethics.

Biomedical ethics

Speaking more broadly, biomedical ethics refers to the application of ethical principles to science, medicine and health care. Nursing ethics therefore relates directly to this (Smith *et al* 1985: 336).

This comprehensive concept reinforces the need, and indeed the urgency, to forge strong interdisciplinary ties.

CLARIFICATION OF ETHICAL CONCEPTS

Every day nurses in clinical practice are faced with situations in which the principles of autonomy, non-maleficence, beneficence, justice and veracity apply. Each of these situations places the nurse in a moral dilemma as the circumstances usually determine her actions and she may not be able to honour these principles.

Autonomy

The principle of autonomy means that patients and clients can expect nurses to provide them with information in such a way that they can understand it and that they will be able to make a decision about the nursing treatment, if any, they prefer, based on this information. 'Nursing treatment requires informed consent just as medical treatment does and for the same ethical reasons' (Smith *et al* 1985: 338).

Non-maleficence

'The principle of non-maleficence requires practitioners not to harm clients intentionally, through lack of knowledge or by negligence. It also requires that practitioners protect clients unable to protect themselves' (Smith et al 1985: 336) (maleficence = harmful).

Beneficence

By this it is meant that patients must be cared for in such a way that possible harm is prevented or removed, and the good of the patient is promoted (Smith et al 1985: 336) (beneficence = doing good).

Justice

Justice refers to fair treatment of patients and the avoidance of discrimination and exploitation (Smith et al 1985: 336).

Veracity

'Veracity requires practitioners to be truthful with clients and maintain confidentiality' (Smith et al 1985: 336). It also implies that the nurse must be truthful in all her dealings.

A PHILOSOPHICAL APPROACH

Ethics has been described as a moral philosophy, so the philosophical approach could be used as a guide to finding answers to questions that arise in nursing practice. Philosophical theory is concerned with understanding the nature of moral judgements and not with providing all the answers.

What use is this approach to the nurse? Do nurses question or discuss moral concepts affecting their everyday nursing practice, such as truth, honesty, loyalty, making promises, conscience, human rights, duty, power, responsibility and accountability, and if not, why not? (after Hockey 1981: 16). The practical implications of such questions are important.

Who must ask these questions related to everyday nursing situations? Surely this affects the practising clinical nurse more than any other, yet she does not appear to be asking such questions herself.

Nurses in top managerial positions do debate these issues and offer solutions which the practising clinical nurses often do not accept because they have not been involved in the decision-making process. If the practising clinical nurse accepted the responsibility for questioning nursing practice according to this approach she would be more likely to implement decisions reached.

The use of this philosophical approach would only benefit the recipients of nursing care and the professional practice of nursing and health care as a whole.

ETHICAL PROBLEMS IN THE PRACTICE OF NURSING

In nursing and medicine, as in so many other walks of life, as man becomes more and more efficient at carrying out technical procedures many new problems develop which only a comparatively short time ago would not have arisen. This section will endeavour to point out some of these problems so that conflicts in the work situation can be understood and the plight of young students caught up in the dilemmas which perplex even more seasoned members of the health team can be treated with sympathy and insight. It is not proposed to offer solutions to problems, that would be beyond the scope of this work, but simply to pose them for the attention of the thoughtful reader.

The sanctity of life

Implied in the nurse's professional code of ethics is the fact that every person who is committed to her care should feel absolutely safe in her hands. The concept of the sanctity of life is tied up with this.

Man, according to the law of nature, has a right to life. He *is*, therefore he *lives*. Nevertheless the life he possesses is transitory, it can be very easily terminated. The present age, where violence seems to be glorified by the media and human life dispensed with seemingly at the drop of a hat, as a means of entertainment, makes it difficult to appreciate the concept that *human life* has a *value*, a *right to reverence*, an *inviolability*, which should be honoured at all times.

The idea that human life should not be destroyed or violated is not universally held; it is not even adhered to by some of the totalitarian regimes of our times. Nevertheless it is part of our Western cultural values, based on the tenets of the Christian religion and Judaism, that human life has 'sanctity'. This follows directly on the Commandment 'Thou shalt not kill' and is based on the belief that because God is the author and giver of life it is wrong for man to destroy it. Man may risk his own health or his life if it is of benefit to another for him to do so, but he has no right to spoil or destroy human life – on the contrary, it is his duty to preserve it.

The non-Christian approach to human life is in many instances the same as the Christian and has been included in declarations of rights, including the Declaration of Geneva adopted by the World Medical Association in 1948 which states: 'I will maintain the utmost respect for human life, from the time of conception; even under threat, I will not use my medical knowledge contrary to the laws of humanity.'

Of course, the laws of many lands also forbid the taking of human life, but as nurses and as colleagues of the physicians we are concerned not only with more than the purely legal aspects, but with the preservation of the life of the human being, remembering that each human being is endowed with human dignity. In respecting the sanctity of his life we are also respecting his human dignity. It is conceivable that in the practice of medicine and of nursing the individual's interpretation of the preservation of the sanctity of life and of human dignity may be different. It is precisely because of the conflict situations that may arise from this and the help and guidance that the young neophyte in the profession requires that this point has been raised.

Young students, from many different backgrounds and with vastly differing experiences of life, often come to nursing with high ideals and with very clear ideas in their minds of right and wrong. They may find that these ideas do not coincide with those of their classmates. They will be confronted with decisions made by others which seem to conflict with what they believe and have hitherto seen as absolute. Grey areas are unkown to them. If those in positions where they are able and expected to give guidance to these students, or even the young, newly registered or enrolled nurses, realise that these problems exist, they will contribute immeasurably to the development of the nurses in question. One cannot solve others' problems for them, but one can help them to find their own answers and solutions. The philosophy of nursing and of life of seasoned practitioners can be an inspiration and an example to the troubled minds of neophytes and help them to develop professional judgement and maturity.

The quality of life

It has been said that man has a right to life and it is the nurse's duty to preserve this. Immediately we concede this we are confronted with another problem, namely: 'Is life, the mere fact of not being clinically dead, the ultimate aim or is the quality of that life important?' Before exploring this question further it might be as well to determine just what 'quality of life' means.

Illness has many facets, and the impact it has on the individual also varies. Illness may be acute or chronic, it may be treatable and either cured completely or partially. Treatment, as far as present knowledge extends, may be futile, that is the illness may be incurable. Illness may or may not be disabling. The mental state of the patient may affect his acceptance or otherwise of illness and treatment.

The patients who suffer from a temporary departure from the state of health, whose condition, whether severe or not, can be cured, are in a different category from the ones who are faced with a chronic disease which is going to alter their life style and which may incapacitate them completely. Although they will not actually be deprived of life as such, the 'quality' or 'degree of excellence' of that life may be seriously affected. People react very differently to chronic illness. This is part of being human. Some will find joy in living, no matter how incapacitated. They will find meaning in what is left to them, while others will not be able to accept a disabling condition no matter how incapacitated. Some will rail against their lot and even seek to terminate it, or implore others to do so.

How can chronic illness affect the quality of life? A few examples may help to clarify this point. Consider the patient who is in need of regular dialysis to sustain life. His whole existence revolves around the machine to which he must be attached at regular intervals. He may well wonder whether life is worth it. The ethical problem occurs when he wants to terminate his life by discontinuing dialysis. His conflict is severe, but the health personnel caring for him also experience conflict. How would they feel in a similar situation? What would they do? Is the life the patient is now forced to live worth it? While not able to participate in the wilful termination of life they can understand the dilemma. Conflicts that arise in the minds of young nurses, and even the more seasoned ones, can readily be understood.

Another case in point might be someone who must take medication regularly in order to stay alive. This is easier than being tied to a machine, for the patient usually controls his own medication. It is imperative that health personnel teach the patient the method of medication and the reasons for taking it so that he is motivated to continue. The health personnel must try to understand the patient's feelings and difficulties so that he can be helped to as normal a life as possible. These feelings and difficulties may be summarised as follows:

- Taking medication regularly makes him 'different' from others and thus 'not normal'. This requires a difficult adjustment.
- He may decide to omit taking a few tablets or injections, thinking that it will not do him any harm.
- He may think that the doctor has made a mistake and so decide to try alternative methods of treatment in a desperate attempt to be healed. Thus herbalists, faith healers, witch-doctors and others are consulted and the medical plan abandoned or followed concurrently, possibly with dire consequences.
- The doctor or nurse who planned his diet or medication programme may fail to take into account individual needs, cultural values and home and work conditions and thus produce an unrealistic plan. The patient may then feel excluded and less inclined to comply with the requirements of the programme.
- Worse still, communication which may seem simple to the communicator may make no sense to the patient and therefore the plan may be neglected or abandoned.

Any member of the health team who deals with a patient whose quality of life is affected by his illness has the moral responsibility to see the total care of the person and not just a fragment thereof as important.

The question posed at the beginning of this section, namely 'Is life, the mere fact of not being clinically dead, the ultimate aim or is the quality of that life important?' can now be considered in the light of the foregoing. Perhaps it is an over-simplification, but, for nurses should not the answer be the following?:

> Because we are committed to the preservation of life it is our duty to sustain that life, but it is up to us to improve the quality of that life at all times, by all the means in our power. We must also understand the conflicts that arise in those patients for whom the quality of life has been adversely affected and our endeavours should be directed to helping them resolve those conflicts.

The quality of life is a subject that can be enlarged upon, *ad infinitum*. That is beyond the scope of this work. One of the ethical problems that arises in the practice of nursing concerns the maintenance of life when the quality is drastically impaired. Awareness that the problem exists and willingness to consider it and help those confronted with it is all that can be expected from such a cursory examination of the subject.

Rights

The public has the right to expect standards of nursing care appropriate to its needs. A tacit social contract between society and the nursing profession is implied and is also necessary for a nurse to be able to meet the health needs of the community. In this way nurses are sanctioned by society to practise their skills in a responsible manner. Many examples of this trust relationship can be quoted from all areas of nursing practice, such as domiciliary midwives who are trusted to carry drugs and to take responsibility for childbirth and primary health care nurses who screen patients, take a full history, do physical examinations, make a diagnosis and prescribe medication up to schedule 4 in certain health care settings.

Ethical problems arise when the rights of the patient and the rights and duties of the doctor or nurse are in conflict. This question has been discussed at great length by medical and nursing ethicists, theologians and philosophers all over the world. These ethical debates have centred around the rights of dying persons.

Truth-telling

It is almost impossible to discuss patients' rights without considering the question of truth-telling. What is the truth? When a patient dies in a hospital ward, in the operating theatre or in an out-patients department the cause of death may not be known, yet his relatives have to be informed. It is usually the responsibility of the nurse to inform the relatives telephonically of the death of the patient. If the death is sudden and unexpected the relatives may appear incredulous and demand to know 'the truth'. If the nurse has no information to offer, especially if there are medico-legal considerations, the relatives may not believe what she has said, and in their agony may accuse her of not telling the truth, of 'hiding' something. This places the nurse in a moral dilemma.

Consider the following situation: A 45-year-old, unemployed male patient and father of three children under the age of three years, admitted to hospital for the treatment of pneumonia, commits suicide by jumping from the fifth floor of the hospital. Who should notify his wife? Should she be told the news telephonically, or should she be asked to come to the hospital immediately? What are her rights in this situation? What if she cannot be contacted telephonically?

In the case of the death of a patient which has been anticipated by the medical team, yet denied by the relatives, should the doctor or nurse inform the relatives at the time of death, or should they ask the relatives to come to the hospital immediately because the patient has taken a bad turn? Should some other person such as the hospital chaplain be involved?

Religious and philosophical views of truth-telling and patient rights

Immanual Kant, a moral philosopher, 'rejects lying as immoral, because if it were universalised it would destroy virtually all moral values that give cohesion and meaning' (C Villa-Vicencio in Benatar 1986: 69). This is one perspective.

Judaism

Another view is that of Jewish thought and law which states that 'human life enjoys an absolute, intrinsic and infinite value. Man is not the owner of his body but merely its custodian, charged to preserve it from any physical harm . . . The doctor's opinion must therefore take precedence over that of the patient, allowing the patient only certain limited rights in such situations, where the medical profession recognises that the chances of saving the patient's life are significantly less than the chances of losing it' (Jakobovitz, I quoted by C Villa-Vicencio in Benatar 1986: 70).

Christianity

The Christian view of death profoundly affects the Christian patient's attitude towards medical and nursing treatment. Generally speaking, to most Christians the concept of the resurrection and of eternal life over-shadows the negative connotation of death held by most Jews. Although it is a view generally held among Christians that death is not to be feared, life on earth is regarded as a gift and ought not to be terminated at will, for instance by suicide. The implication of this for nurses is that if a Christian unsuccessfully attempts to commit suicide, he or she may have to work through a lot of guilt afterwards. Nurses and doctors who are not of this faith ought to be aware of this possibility.

Roman Catholicism

This form of Christianity has some differing points of view of which a nurse should be aware. A Roman Catholic view of the situation is that

> both the views of the doctor and the patient are pertinent in the healing process, and the patient, wherever possible, ought to be allowed to exercise his or her freedom to decide what course of healing ought to be followed. If it is not possible for doctor or patient to agree, in the course of *normal* medical practice, Soane argues that the doctor, as the person responsible for the medical process, has a right to override the wish of the patient (Brendan Soane, as quoted by C Villa-Vicencio in Benatar 1986: 70).

Yet, in extraordinary situations, the patient may refuse treatment if, in the opinion of the doctor, the prescribed treatment merely prolongs an untenable situation. It would appear, then, that it ought to be common practice for patients of the Roman Catholic persuasion to expect doctors to consult them about the treatment programme. Doctors and nurses of this faith may expect their colleagues to adhere to the same values as they do. If they do not, this may lead to conflict.

Buddhism

To a Buddhist 'the death of a human being occurs when he is volitionally dead'. Therefore it is said that if a person is no longer able to make a decision, there is no real point in keeping him alive (Louis van Loon, as quoted by C Villa-Vicencio in Benatar 1986: 71). It would appear then, that the overriding consideration here is the quality of life.

The Islamic faith

This faith believes 'that man has been created by God, that life is a gift from God (not an accident) and man is its steward . . . the doctor is bound to promote health and life, to strive actively against any power which undermines the sanctity of the human being, his life and his person' (Najaar, A, in Benatar 1985: 30). The emphasis is on *care* rather than treatment, and that the doctor's, the patient's and the family's decisions regarding cost, circumstances and so on will determine the extent and nature of care. The dying person has the right to choose where he wishes to spend his final days – this will often be at home with his family. Euthanasia is rejected completely and abortion is acceptable only if the mother's life is in danger.

It is important for nurses to be aware of these different religious and philosophical attitudes to life and death and the rights of patients, and to think about them, as this knowledge influences the nurse-patient and nurse-doctor relationship. It also enables the nurse to understand the patient's perception of his or her rights as an individual, especially as these rights are affected by medical treatment programmes.

Power

The word 'power' usually has a negative connotation in present day Western society, but power can also be regarded as a professional privilege which should be honoured by health care professionals. Power can be defined as the ability to do or act, delegated authority, capacity for exerting force (*Concise Oxford Dictionary*, 4th ed). It can thus be seen that the word 'power' has wide application and is certainly not a negative concept, except perhaps in the sense of 'exerting force'.

The evolving role of the nurse

In South Africa, the changing health care needs of the various communities, the maldistribution of medical practitioners and the subsequent evolution of nursing practice to meet these needs has led to the concomitant evolving role of the nurse.

The traditional image of the nurse in England was of a carer of the sick, content to allow others to make decisions for her. This image is rapidly changing and the modern nurse is emerging as an intelligent, questioning professional facing a major challenge, and her responsibility is closely connected with a legal, moral and ethical liability. She can only meet this challenge if there is an improvement in nurse-education on law and ethics and she is no longer regarded as a pair of hands (Dixon 1982: 301).

This new image of the nurse is already well-entrenched in the health care services in South Africa.

A more relevant curriculum, at both basic and post-basic level, which includes university programmes, has equipped the professional nurse for the additional responsibilities and for independent practice. This applies particularly to primary health care settings, some of which are manned almost exclusively by specially trained primary health care nurses. This type of nursing practice has, by implication and in reality, given the nurse power in these situations. Power in this context can never be absolute by virtue of the ethical constraints within which the professional nurse practises.

Power sharing

In the discussions that follow on the advances made in medical technology, organ transplantation and ethanasia, reference has been made, directly and indirectly, to the concept power.

Nurses do not work in isolation, but as part of a team. 'In the age of high technology, nurses are beginning to recognise the nexus between knowledge and power, and, in the light of this recognition, to question the role relationship between nurses and other health professionals' (Brewer, A, 1983, as quoted by Woodruff 1985: 298). This role relationship implies a sharing of this privileged professional power. In certian countries professional interdisciplinary battles are raging over questions of power and authority, whereas in South Africa this has not become an issue. As stated earlier, nursing ethical and legal codes clearly delineate the scope of nursing practice that should prevent such conflict. The onus is on each professional nurse to practise her skills with competence, insight and vision in order to maintain an acceptable standard of practice.

This power must be shared *with* clients and patients because of the tacit agreement between society and the nursing profession. The public has become well-informed about health care matters via the mass media and is more aware of the right to health than ever before. Therefore members of the public will no longer tolerate a situation where health care providers have power *over* them.

Abuse of power

It is imperative for professional nurses to honour the privilege bestowed on them. They must exercise such power within the health care services and not abuse it, since it affects patients and colleagues. Nurse-nurse loyalty must be respected and victimisation within the professional ranks must be avoided.

Where it exists, it must be exposed and dealt with. Existing nursing legislation oils the wheels of the profession, ensuring a therapeutic environment for patients and one that is conducive to professional growth. It also prevents exploitation and emphasises the fact that the nurse's first responsibility is to the patient.

CONFLICTS IN THE WORK SITUATION

Medical power has become so great that ethical problems are inevitable and conflicts in the work situation will arise. Some of these will be discussed here.

Medical technology

Machines

A person may be kept 'alive', that is with some degree of biological functioning, for long periods with the aid of various life-support machines. These machines perform functions such as respiration (ventilators) and maintaining an adequate arterial blood pressure (intra-aortic balloon counterpulsation pumps) and a physiologically acceptable blood chemistry (dialyzers). Depending on the condition of the patient, the use of these machines may be temporary and the duration of treatment short. However, an ethical problem arises when a decision has to be made as to whether to preserve the life of a patient for whom the chances of survival are poor or for whom the quality of life will be severely impaired. 'While the work in an intensive care unit can be exciting and rewarding when there is hope to save the life of a person, it may become absurd when there is no hope of cure and when the prescribed treatment interferes with a last stage of life spent in peace, comfort, dignity and close contact with loved ones' (Poletti 1985: 330).

Decisions concerning prolongation of life are fraught with anguish for the family. On the one hand there is the desire to see the end of the agony, but on the other there is the desire to postpone the moment of death. Nurses ought to be aware of the dilemma experienced by relatives and try to be understanding, sympathetic and compassionate. They ought to be able to assess the strengths of the family and in this way to help family members to cope with the situation by utilising the potential or overt strengths of each of the family members.

The cost factor

Another aspect of technology to be considered is the cost factor. Machines are, to a varying degree, extremely expensive to acquire, to maintain and to operate. If financial provision is such that institutions have as much money as they need, then the purchase of expensive equipment is no problem, but where financial resources are limited the allocation of these resources according to the priorities of health needs will have to be carefully considered. The provision of health care services that will benefit the common good rather than benefiting the good of the few, that is the utilitarian approach, is currently a much debated issue worldwide. An ethical problem arises when only one machine is available for the treatment of two or more patients needing the treatment. Such a situation poses a grave moral dilemma for the doctor which is shared by the nurse. Although the decision is not the nurses's, her emotional conflict and the difficulty she may have in accepting decisions must be understood. The nurse, in turn, must also be able to understand the doctor's problems and be ready to support him in his extremely difficult task.

The ageing population

Technology and improved health care services have contributed to another problem faced by modern society, that of longevity and therefore an ever-increasing aged population with its specific health-related problems. Pneumonia, for example, used to be called 'the friend of the aged. Taken off by it in an acute, short, not often painful illness, the old man escapes those "cold gradations of decay" so distressing to himself and to his friends' (Osler, WO, as in Hirschfeld, MJ 1985: 320). 'But the old man's friend is dead, a victim of medical progress. Pharmacological and technological advances extending life have become methods of extending disease as well. The course of senile brain disease has been extended from an average of three to over twelve years' (Gruenberg EM, *et al* in Hirschfeld, MJ 1985: 320).

The increased need for care of geriatric patients has made greater calls on nursing care and has even necessitated the introduction of a specialised nursing course to meet the needs of patients from this group.

Computers

The use of computers in health care institutions has made the problem of confidentiality more difficult. What was once regarded as privileged communication, that is 'information given to a professional person such as a physician, nurse or social worker' is now accessible to non-professional staff members as computerised information (Kozier *et al* 1982: 14).

The implication for nursing is that nurses have to become computer literate. This is easier for the neophyte, who often comes from school already used to this form of technology. It poses problems for the older members of the profession, who may need intensive in-service education to function in this new field.

Computers can make health care more efficient and must be seen as an adjunct to personal care and not as a replacement for it. The confidentiality aspect must be guarded against as far as this is humanly possible. As a patient advocate the nurse should be aware of the existence of systems whereby information can be coded so that access is less readily available to all. Where such a system is not yet in use the nurse has a duty to point out the need for one.

The search for clinical knowledge

Because of the dynamic nature of nursing and medicine the search for clinical knowledge continues unabated. This includes research into technology and it is in this area of clinical practice that caution is necessary. Nurses are taught to use technology to facilitate nursing practice, especially in intensive care units, but this has ethical implications. If nurses rely too heavily on technology-based criteria to guide their decisions with regard to patient care there is the danger that they may lose their clinical observation skills. These skills require the use of the nurse's senses of sight, hearing, smell and touch in assessing a patient's condition. In this respect it must again be emphasised that the nurse's first responsibility is to the patient.

Organ transplantation

The transplantation of certain human organs such as the heart, lungs, kidney, liver and pancreas with varying degrees of success has raised ethical questions. Recently, the implantation of an artificial heart has also been undertaken.

Financial implications

Most transplantation programmes are undertaken at great cost to the health care institution or to the patient, depending on where in the world the operation is performed. In South Africa the cost is to the institution rather than to the patient, since this service is offered by State hospitals only. This may change with increased privatisation of medical services in South Africa. 'Whilst the State or other organization may bear the cost of the operation and post-operative care, the facilities available to maintain the recipient awaiting transplantation and his family may be inadequate' (Commerford, PJ as quoted in Cooper and Lanza 1984: 19). The cost of transplantation programmes, which includes the hidden costs of the waiting period, poses ethical questions in terms of the prudent allocation of scarce resources.

Selection of the recipient

When a patient is considered for transplantation surgery no major contra-indications must be detected if he is to be accepted. The surgeon must obtain *informed* consent, which means that the patient must understand 'the nature of the treatment offered, the potential benefits, as well as the necessity of prolonged post-operative hospitalization, follow-up, and the hazards associated with immuno-suppression' (Commerford, PJ, as quoted in Cooper and Lanza 1984: 16).

This is an extremely difficult period for the patient emotionally and psychologically. He will already be physically compromised, since these patients nearly always have a chronic disease. Both he and his family will need constant reassurance, encouragement and support. Patients in this situation often turn to sub-professional nurses or even domestic staff for comfort and advice. This may pose ethical problems for professional nurses and for doctors, but it emphasises the need for an appreciation of the very real fear experienced by patients in these circumstances.

Preparation of the family

It has been well documented that a strong supportive family considerably assists the patient to adjust and to cope with the post-operative period. In this respect the nurse has a major role to play in enabling the family to adjust to the changed roles precipitated by the illness. She can help the patient to gain insight into his role as a patient without relinquishing the roles of husband, boyfriend, brother, son, professional person or friend, although these roles may already have been modified because of the illness. The nurse can be a great support to the family if she is able to assess and utilise family strengths, such as good communication between family members and outsiders, understanding, tolerance, humour, empathy, love, support and taking and maintaining an interest in the patient and in his 'sick world'.

Selection and management of the donor

The question of organ donation remains a sensitive issue. This may be so because of misconceptions or unrealistic fears about the donation of organs in the minds of laymen. Attitudes also vary according to cultural beliefs, religious views, levels of knowledge, literacy and the personal preferences of various cultural groups.

For transplant purposes, kidneys and bone marrow may be obtained from live donors or from cadavers. Today it is also possible to remove and preserve organs for short periods in tissue banks.

Cadaver donation

It is not an easy task to approach bereaved relatives for the purpose of obtaining consent for the removal of organs for transplant surgery. 'For the layman it is still a macabre concept that the heart can be beating when doctors speak of death. They may not be able to grasp this concept, and this possibility should be respected, particularly when such understanding has to occur across cultural dividing lines' (De Villiers, JC, as quoted in Cooper and Lanza 1984: 32). Expert counselling skills, compassion and wisdom are required in such situations. To make this easier for all concerned, medic alert discs or donor cards should be worn on the person of a voluntary donor of organs at all times.

Cadaver donation is considered only after the establishment of the fact of brain death. The criteria for brain death can be found in Appendix E. In order to preserve the organs of the donor in the most satisfactory condition for transplant surgery, mechanical ventilation of the donor is continued after brain death has been established. The potential legal and ethical problems anticipated by the medical profession after the performance of the first human heart transplant were eliminated with the publication of the Declaration of Sydney in 1968, in which the World Medical Association stated that two or more doctors should determine the moment of death, and that these doctors must be independent of the transplant team (Scorer and Wing 1979: 194). When organs are available for transplantation doctors are faced with the difficult decision as to who the recipient will be, although this problem has been eliminated to a large extent by the tissue and blood compatibility tests that are performed pre-operatively. These tests narrow the range of options, as the recipient and the donor must be histocompatible. Nevertheless, the human element in the ethical dilemma of having to make a decision between two equally suitable recipients cannot be forgotten.

Living donors

The living donor of a kidney is often closely related to the recipient, since the chances of successful transplantation are so much greater in these circumstances. Here the supportive role of the nurse cannot be stressed enough. She should encourage both the donor and the recipient to express their fears, uncertainties and anxieties to her and possibly also to each other. Feelings of guilt on the part of the donor in the case of an unsuccessful operation must be avoided, or, if evident, dealt with in a sensitive manner.

Obtaining consent for donation of organs

The most important legal consideration of all transplant operations is that of valid consent. *The Human Tissue Act* (No 65 of 1983) deals with the removal of human tissue for transplantation purposes. This Act specifically makes provision for the following legal requirements:

- [ ] certification of the fact of death
- [ ] who may donate
- [ ] who the donee may be
- [ ] who is required to give authority for the removal of the donated heart or kidney
- [ ] certain administrative matters pertaining to such donation and use (Cooper *et al* 1982: 837).

Selling organs

A highly controversial topic is whether a person should be allowed to sell his organs for donation. This practice has been condemned by leading transplantation societies. Such a practice is open to abuse.

Career opportunities resulting from transplantation surgery

Transplantation surgery has opened up new career opportunities for nurses. In some of the transplant centres in South Africa posts have been created for nursing transplant coordinators, whose main function is the coordination of the activities between the transplant services and nursing staff caring for potential donors at the base and neighbouring hospitals. (Cooper *et al* 1982: 934).

Euthanasia

This word is used so much in the public media these days that brief attention to it will not be out of place.

The term 'euthanasia' is derived from the Greek *eu* (well) and *thanotos* (death), meaning a 'well', 'good' or 'easy' death. Although he knows that death is inevitable, man tends to shy away from acknowledging this fact. Death always happens to 'someone else'. There is fear of death, but perhaps even greater is the fear of the pain and suffering that often accompanies death. Thus an easy, painless death is the wish of all, and this is what the term euthanasia really means.

Nevertheless, in the context of everyday language usage it has come to be linked with *mercy killing*, which is another matter altogether. Modern medicine has made prolongation of life by mechancial means possible. (This has already been discussed under 'Quality of life'.) The avoidance of actual physical death even though 'brain death' may have occurred has made it possible to prolong life beyond what many people consider necessary.

Permitting death to occur earlier than would be the case if the patient were attached to life-support machines or subjected to heroic lifesaving measures is often referred to as *passive euthanasia*. There are four relatively common situations in which the problem of whether to *permit* death may arise and internal conflicts may be experienced by those who are committed to the care of such patients. This applies particularly to young students who have close, physical contact with patients. The areas in which these problems arise are the following:

☐ Continued life support by artificial means for those with extensive brain damage

☐ Continued treatment, other than that ensuring freedom from pain and general comfort for patients suffering from terminal illnesses

☐ Indiscriminate emergency resuscitation for cardiac arrest

☐ Deciding which patient to treat when facilities, personnel, etc make it possible to treat only a limited number.

In the first instance it is not the nurse's decision to switch off machines. Nevertheless, as a feeling, thinking member of society and as a citizen of the world she will have views on the subject, especially as she is in close contact with the patient, his relatives and friends, often over quite a long period of time.

In the second area mentioned *the decision whether to continue specific, often heroic, treatment in 'hopeless' cases* is often one for the patient himself. Today many thinking persons are signing the 'Living Will', wherein they state that under certain conditions they do not wish to have their lives prolonged by 'heroic' measures when there is no hope of recovery. With more emphasis on special units for the care of the terminally ill, where peace of mind and alleviation of unpleasant symptoms are all-important, the nurse with special aptitudes for this type of nursing may find her niche. The patient who has accepted the inevitability of death will nevertheless need support and understanding, as will his relatives and friends, for they are the ones who will be left behind after the patient has gone. Another factor which merits consideration here, for it may cloud the emotional reactions of nurses, is whether it is justified to give medications which may shorten life, but will relieve suffering. Again the nurse does not prescribe the treatment or otherwise, but she administers it and therefore may have conflicting thoughts about it.

The third problem area is that of *indiscriminate emergency resuscitation* after cardiac arrest. Speed is of the essence here and will affect the decision, for it is an established fact that failure to restore circulation to the cells of the brain within a few moments will result in irreparable cerebral damage. Attempts to resuscitate may thus be abandoned if there is no rapid response and may not even be made if the time lag between the arrest and the possibility of treatment has been too great. Decisions of this sort are not easily made; the scientific basis for this must be clearly understood. It is one thing to defibrillate a patient already attached to a monitor in an intensive care unit if sudden cardiac arrest should occur, but quite another to attempt to restart a heart in a casualty department when the patient arrested some time before. Nevertheless nurses, especially those who are very new to the profession, may feel that 'not enough was done', or 'nothing was done' in the latter case, without perceiving why this was so. The nurse will also have to deal with shocked members of the family confronted with such a situation.

A *coding system for resuscitation* is used in certain countries. Such a coding system, known to all members of the health team, obviates the need for discussion of the decision to resuscitate at the bedside within earshot of relatives or other patients, or even of the patient himself. As it is generally agreed that hearing is the last sense to be lost, it would seem kind to spare the patient the possibility of hearing and understanding the details of this ethical decision. To some professionals the use of a coding system may be quite unacceptable. However, if such ethical decisions are based on the *art* with which medicine is practised, that is the 'wisdom, prudence, compassion, patience, sensitivity to ethical issues and devotion with which physicians apply their scientific knowledge to the care of their patients', then it would seem that a coding system for resuscitation is a humane approach to patient care (Benatar 1986: 10).

The fourth problem area arises in *disaster situations involving large numbers of persons,* where 'triage officers' have the onerous and often unpleasant task of deciding which of the casualties are most likely to benefit from emergency treatment, and of establishing priorities. The people actually giving the treatment must not be involved in this decision making, for the conflicts will be too great. Nurses involved in receiving and caring for the casualties will obviously have conflicting emotions regarding the establishment of priorities. They need to understand the difficult decisions made by triage officers, who have to decide, for instance, whether sending a casualty with little hope of recovery for treatment will not delay the care of one with a better chance so much that he also becomes as ill as the first one. Thus two lives are lost when one might have been saved.

The other aspect of euthanasia, active 'mercy-killing', is more clear-cut. In our country, and in many others, it is illegal and cannot be condoned no matter how sympathetically one may feel towards it. It cannot be overemphasised that *the nurse is committed to sustain human life and to ameliorate suffering*. There is a *tremendous trust relationship between the nurse and the patient* as a result of the tacit contract between society and the nursing profession. The patient must feel completely safe in the hands of any nurse responsible for his care. This is an ethical concept which must be preseved no matter what emotional overtones enter into the matter. Much has been written and said on this subject, much more will be written and spoken in the future.

Religious attitudes must also be taken into consideration. The purpose of this short section on euthanasia is to point out that conflicts in the minds of nurses and other members of the health team, as well as of patients and their loved ones, will occur and should be dealt with with sympathy, understanding and support. Nurses need to clarify their own thoughts and philosophies and to be able to present to those committed to their care an image of a person who is worthy of such trust, one who will help and support those in need of such support in life and, until death, will sustain that life as a sacred trust while affording the patient alleviation of unnecessary suffering and consideration as a bearer of human dignity.

Treatment: must one because one can?

This problem is tied up with all the other problems. In this situation one is confronted not only with resuscitation or life-support problems, but with the question of whether or not it is morally right or ethical to carry out certain forms of treatment just because the knowledge and expertise is available. Should we do something to a patient just because we can do it? It must be remembered that the patient has the right of refusal. 'Consent' is necessary, but there are times when it may be necessary for the nurse to use a degree of persuasion or even coercion in order to achieve a result.

A case in point would be assisting to rehabilitate an amputee. Getting him out of bed, to exercise, fitting an artificial limb and making the patient use it may require some coercion. Is this always justified? Consider the case of the elderly amputee who has lost both legs as a result of diabetic gangrene. It is generally considered desirable to get him as mobile as possible, but is it morally right to coerce him into the use of artificial limbs which may, in any case, cause breakdown of tissue and lead to falls and a great deal of suffering? Of course this will depend on the patient, but it merits consideration. Must one continue with these methods just because one can? The answer to the question cannot be given. It does present a moral dilemma.

Much more clear-cut would be the decision to encourage and even coerce into action a young amputee who has lost both legs in a motor accident. He may rail against his fate, refuse to cooperate and generally cause problems, but life for him has a different potential if he can only be brought to a realisation of its possibilities and it would be wrong not to apply pressure towards attaining full mobility.

Such a dilemma confronting a physician might be whether to actively treat the pneumonia of a patient suffering from terminal malignant disease, or merely to alleviate the symptoms. Again the decision is not the nurse's, but she will be intimately linked with its consequences. Many other similar instances could be quoted, but it is sufficient to point out that such ethical dilemmas exist in the work situation. It is important to realise that actions are not always either *only good* or *only bad*. They may include elements of both and there are few, if any, clear-cut answers.

The only possible approach is to weigh up the situations according to the information available and try to find a solution that will bring the maximum good to the recipient of care within the legal and ethical codes governing the profession.

Genetics

Some contemporary ethical issues which should receive attention include genetics and genetic engineering.

NV Rothwell (1977: 1) says that genetics is the science which studies 'the nature of hereditary material, how it is transmitted, how it interacts with the environment to bring about an effect on a cell or an individual'. In recent years this particular science has advanced dramatically. Public interest in and awareness of genetics and genetic counselling services have grown apace. The call for genetic counselling in primary prevention, where there is a possibility of genetic malformation or disease, is increasing. More and more nurses are being employed in genetics clinics and need to be made aware of the type of work involved so that they are able to consider the ethical problems that may arise and examine their own attitudes to this field of work. Genetic counselling prior to pregnancy and birth is becoming more prevalent. The pre-natal diagnosis of genetic defects may involve the termination of a pregnancy. It must be stressed that genetic counselling leaves the choice to the parents, but it may still present a conflict situation for nurses, who must also have freedom of choice with regard to working in such a service.

Genetic engineering

Genetic engineering is an even more controversial subject, and although research has been undertaken it is still too early to say how far this aspect of genetics has progressed or what the ultimate possibilities or implications may be. Dramatic beneficial progress is being made.

Changing the genetic structure of a potential human being still has a 'science-fiction' image, but it is as well that nurses are aware of such possibilities and of the ethical problems that may arise. Where should the line be drawn?

Abortion

This is an area in which conflict may arise. An abortion is generally taken to be 'the interruption of pregnancy before the 28th week of gestation, after which period the fetus is viable (capable of a separate existence)' (Myles 1981: 158).

Abortion may occur spontaneously as a result of maternal disease, the effect of some drugs on the mother, ABO incompatibility between the mother and embryo, trauma, an incompetent cervix, fibrous tumours of the uterus and implantation of the ovum in the lower uterine segment, as well as abnormal foetal development. An abortion that arises from these causes should not present ethical problems. Concern for the mental and physical state of the mother should be the primary concern of the nurse.

Termination of pregnancy by taking deliberate measures is legally controlled by the *Abortion and Sterilisation Act*, 1975 (Act 2 of 1975). As a method of getting rid of an unwanted pregnancy, it is illegal in South Africa. The legal requirements for an abortion are the following:

☐ Where the continued pregnancy endangers the life of a woman
☐ Where the continued pregnancy constitutes a serious threat to a woman's physical health
☐ Where the continued pregnancy constitutes a serious threat to a woman's mental health and is of such a nature as to create the danger of permanent damage to her health and the abortion is necessary to ensure her mental health
☐ Where there exists a serious risk that the child to be born will suffer from a physical or mental defect of such a nature that he will be irreparably seriously handicapped
☐ Where the foetus was conceived in consequence of rape
☐ Where the foetus was conceived in incest
☐ Where the foetus was conceived in unlawful carnal intercourse with a female idiot or imbecile.

Despite the legality of some abortions a nurse may find the concept contrary to her religious beliefs. No nurse can be forced to participate in an abortion, no matter how legal, if it is against her beliefs and principles. Such a nurse must make her standpoint known to nursing management in all cases where she is likely to be called upon to assist in an abortion. Refusal to participate does not absolve her from care of the patient after an abortion. It is completely wrong for any nurse, for anyone indeed, to take part in *illegal* abortions. Abortion on demand is *not legal*, no matter how much emotional pity for a pregnant woman there may be. Nurses must know the legal aspects of abortion; students should be aware of the ethical problems involved and debate the subject during the course of their preparation for the role of professional nurse.

Family planning (birth or population control)

The findings of the Science Committee of the President's Council on Demographic Trends, published in 1983, revealed the fact that South Africa could support a population of only 80 million in terms of non-renewable resources (Rip *et al* 1986: 70).

The factors that influence population growth are economic development, adult literacy and formal education, health and medical services, social and family structures and functions, urbanisation and family planning programmes. Nurses have an important role to play in each of these areas and at national policy-making level in promoting healthy lifestyles for South African citizens and preventing disease and an unprecedented population increase, which could compound the problem of over-population and its concomitant social evils. The prediction that South Africa will have a population of 180 million by the year 2020, a mere 33 years away, is a matter of grave concern according to Rip *et al* (1986: 70). An important step in population control was the introduction of the Population Development Programme to supplement the existing family planning programme.

Family planning can also be a conflict area, for there are some religious and cultural groups that believe that the only acceptable method of preventing pregnancy is abstinence from sexual intercourse. This subject should be thoroughly explained and debated so that nurses can clarify their feelings and decide for themselves whether they will take part in such programmes.

A nurse has the right to withdraw from programmes or actions that are not ethically acceptable to her. All the methods used for family planning should be known to her, from oral and injectable contraceptives, intrauterine devices, the diaphragm, the condom and the use of spermicidal agents, to sterilisation of the male or female, but actual participation in such a programme is a matter of individual conscience.

The handling of products of conception

These may include an aborted foetus, placenta, etc. The nurse must be conversant with cultural practices regarding the disposal of the products of conception, which extends to the disposal of the placenta after birth. It is an ethical responsibility to know what is expected in these cases and to comply with special requirements, unless some definite health hazard is involved. The feelings and beliefs of patients and clients must be respected. The different ethnic practices and religious observances are part of the study of the ethos and thus also of the ethical aspects of nursing.

Artificial insemination – in vitro fertilisation (test-tube babies) and similar procedures; surrogate mothers

Today these techniques are all possible. Artificial insemination of a woman with her husband's semen is often acceptable to certain groups, while artificial insemination with donor semen may not be. To others, neither is acceptable. Again, *both* methods may find acceptance in the eyes of some. Besides legal components, the moral and religious views differ. Sterilisation of an ovum outside the body and even the freezing of fertilised ova for future implantation in the uterus is another technique being practised. Therefore, women can be fertilised with the stored semen of husbands who have died. There are certain legal implications attached to such procedures which should be considered. Nurses need to be well-informed about such matters and therefore able to make their own ethical decisions.

The implantation of a fertilised ovum in a surrogate mother, who then bears the child for the genetic mother, is also possible. This poses even more ethical, religious and legal problems which should also be carefully investigated and discussed from all angles so that nurses can arrive at their own views and make their own decisions based on knowledge and understanding.

As science and technology become more and more advanced, more and more 'difficult' situations, which require careful consideration each time they present themselves, will arise.

* * *

Other problems that may crop up in nursing practice and of which the nurse must be aware include child abuse, spouse battering, geriatric abuse, adolescent sexuality, the abnormal neonate, the brain-damaged child, the brain-damaged adult and drug abuse. The nurse, as a caring human being, will see many facets of all of the above. She may be torn between what she feels and what she believes. Her attitude must be non-judgemental. When in doubt she must be able to confide in a trusted colleague who, by allowing her to express her doubts, fears and what she has observed, can help her to awareness of the courses of action open to her so that she can come to a decision for herself.

Ethical considerations related to research

Nurses are often involved in research and it is appropriate that a few words should be devoted to this subject.

Clinical research is the use of the experimental method and observation to study disease symptoms, patterns and processes as they occur in sick people. The aim of this research, or *careful search and inquiry into*, is to acquire new knowledge about disease, its treatment and man's reponse to treatment for the ultimate benefit of not only the specific patient concerned, but also future possible patients. Research may include an element of danger and may cause the patient anxiety and discomfort.

If diagnostic procedures are included in the definition of research then the possibility of injury or even death cannot be entirely excluded. Nevertheless, without research to enable us to treat the patient of tomorrow more effectively than it is possible to treat the patient of today, there can be no progress. Doctors have a moral (ethical) responsibility to observe and evaluate alternative methods of treatment and to search for more knowledge so as to improve practice. A draft code of ethics on human experimentation was drawn up by the World Medical Association in 1962. It was revised and accepted at the meeting of the World Medical Association in June 1964 and is known as the Declaration of Helsinki.

Ethical guidelines

The doctor's mission is to safeguard the health of the people. His knowledge and conscience are dedicated to the fulfilment of this mission.

'The Declaration of Geneva of the World Medical Association binds the doctor with the words "The health of my patient will be my first consideration;" and the International Code of Medical Ethics declares that "Any act or advice which could weaken physical or mental resistance of a human being may be used only in his interest"' (Scorer and Wing 1979: 193). See Appendix F for details of the Declaration of Geneva and the Declaration of Helsinki.

Nursing research

Research is increasingly becoming a part of the world of nursing. In the unit situation nurses are constantly participating in clinical trials and in medical research projects where, for the most part, they act as research assistants. The ultimate aim of research in nursing is to improve health care through the process of nursing. Bearing this in mind nurses must initiate, undertake and participate in nursing research. If they undertake nursing research with open minds, with interest and enthusiasm, and in such a way that it is subject to the legal and ethical considerations applicable to any form of research into health care, much that is valuable will be achieved. Nurses need to know how to think and reason in a logical way; they must be able to come to valid conclusions based on sound knowledge, examination of a problem and careful investigation. Nurses are constantly faced with the need to make decisions based on knowledge and a summing up of the elements of the situation, that is on the conclusions arrived at in a scientific manner, even if the steps are rapid and take place mentally. Nurses do not 'guess' what they must do — they do not rely only on 'intuition', but on scientific, orderly thinking.

In the past nursing research has been restricted to the work done by nurses undertaking a research project for post-graduate study and to those investigating administrative or organisational problems. The South African Nursing Association has recognised the need for research and has established a research division at its headquarters in Pretoria, with a research officer on the staff.

Where does the nurse stand? The *Declaration of Helsinki* provides useful guidelines for the nurse with regard to professional attitudes based on sound ethical concepts. Participation in many research projects may involve the nurse in nothing more spectacular than the routine collection of specimens or the observation and notation of simple data. At other times it may be far more complex and involve risks to the patient. The nurse's participation may include helping to motivate the patient to submit to research, which may cause concern to the individual nurse. Doubts as to whether she is really justified in motivating the patient in such circumstances may arise.

Clinical reasearch must be carried out meticulously. Accurate observation and reporting is essential if results are to be obtained. Carelessness cannot be tolerated.

When nurses are doing independent research into nursing they are governed by their code of professional ethics. Any ethical problems involved in performing nursing research should be resolved within this framework. The nurse is concerned with a unique type of service to those with special needs. Observation is part of her stock in trade, as is accurate recording of findings. She applies them as carefully in routine research procedures as she does in her usual patient care record-keeping.

The health care professional of today is faced with many more complex issues requiring decision making than has ever been the case in the history of medicine, nursing or allied disciplines. Research, with all it implies, has solved many problems and made available many methods of treatment that were formerly unknown. At the same time it has created new ethical problems besides those inherent in the research process. The need for the nurse to give careful consideration to all aspects mentioned in this short section on the ethical basis of the profession of nursing cannot be over-emphasised, and should form an integral part of the education of the professional nurse. Ethical concepts must be part of all teaching and learning in the profession of nursing.

7 The concept 'duty'

Duty is used so frequently with regard to nursing that, although it is largely an ethical concept, it has been felt necessary to devote a separate chapter to the subject.

Phrases such as 'it is your duty to do so', 'do your duty' and 'she neglected her duty' are heard frequently, but so also are terms like 'duty-time', 'spells of duty', 'on-duty' and 'off-duty'. 'Duty' can also mean a tax levied on goods, so that everyone is familiar with terms such as 'duty-free', 'customs duty' and 'death-duty'. A 'duty' can also be 'owed to someone'.

From this one can see that the phrase, 'it is your duty to' means 'it is your moral obligation to', while 'neglect of duty' means 'neglect of what one is bound to do', and terms like 'duty-time' (time owed to service or to an employer) 'on-duty' (while giving service owed) are also readily understood.

What, then, is a nurse's 'duty' and to whom does she owe this 'duty'? A duty, according to the definition already examined, means 'that which is owed', be it service, care, loyalty, respect, tax or time. It is the moral necessity to do or to omit to do something, what one ought or ought not to do. The nurse, governed by her professional code of ethics and the basic principles of professional practice in nursing, should by this time have a fair idea of what she 'ought' or 'ought not' to do. At the same time it would be well for her to examine carefully those to whom she owes a duty and to realise that at some time or other there is likely to be a 'conflict of duty' which she alone will be capable of resolving.

DUTY TO FELLOW MEN

Because of the tremendous service motive underlying their professional practice, nurses owe a duty to their fellow men in perhaps larger measure than some other categories of worker. The various groups with which nurses are concerned are the following:

Clients or patients

In the modern concept of health care, those involved in its delivery are as concerned with keeping people healthy as with the treatment of disease when it occurs. This fits in, too, with the definition of nursing given in chapter 1. The term *client* has come into use for those receiving service of a preventive or promotive nature from health care personnel and *patient* is reserved for those who are actually suffering from disease or deformity (infirmity). Thus a *client* may become a *patient* and a *patient* a *client*. Both are recipients of care and the nurse owes a duty to both.

It follows that her duty to her clients or patients will embrace the highest standards of professional competence and practice so that she owes it to them to keep up to date, be technically competent, be skilled at observation, notation and reporting and be ready to provide quality care or to ensure that those for whom she is responsible give quality nursing care at all times. The exercise of sound professional judgement in carrying out the independent functions of a professional nurse as well as the dependent function for the benefit of her clients or patients is a *sine qua non* for her duty to these human beings, her fellow men.

In being concerned with clients and patients the nurse also has a duty to those nearest and dearest to them. A client or patient does not exist in isolation and often the success of a preventive, promotive or therapeutic programme depends on the cooperation of others. Duty to clients and patients implies an awareness of their needs. Observation is the basis of this, with knowledge and skill to interpret what is observed so that action may be instigated. A nurse may never make the excuses 'I did not notice' and 'I did not know', for she *should*, as part of her *duty*, have noticed and *should have known*, or at least found out if there was doubt in her mind.

The nurse's moral obligation or duty to her clients or patients is to promote, as far as is humanly possible, their total well-being in the circumstances in which they find themselves. No two clients or patients will react in quite the same way to the same conditions, for no two conditions will ever be exactly the same. The duty of the nurse is to apply the nursing process by assessing needs, planning action, implementing the plan, evaluating and recording results and reassessing needs. This can be done only when the nurse sees her duty to her clients and patients as embracing:

- *care* and *concern* for the total well-being of clients/patients
- *knowledge* and understanding of needs and ways of meeting these
- *cooperation* of and with clients/patients, their family and friends and members of the health team
- *communication* between the client/patient and all persons or categories of workers concerned with his well-being
- *consideration* for human worth and dignity
- *curiosity* so that she never stops learning
- *complete disregard* for the race, colour, creed or political or economic status of a client/patient in her care, except where cultural factors influence disease patterns and treatment.

Colleagues

The nurse's colleagues in the health care delivery team are many and varied. They include other nurses, physicians, paramedical workers, social workers, dieticians and many more.

The nurse owes a duty to them all. She usually acts as coordinator of all the services rendered to the client or patient who is, or should be, the concern of the whole team and not only the individual practitioner. She owes to these colleagues loyalty, cooperation, giving of her best in nursing care, clear and accurate reporting, consultation and assistance. In some circumstances help and guidance may be necessary. Modern health care is a team effort. The nurse is an important member of the team, but not the only member. To be cheerful and willing and working together is the duty of all members of the team, but the overriding concern is for the welfare of the client/patient.

Working amicably with colleagues does not mean a lowering of standards in order to 'give in' to another or to have 'peace at any price'. *Good must be done, and be seen to be done, for others by all.* Compromise may be the only solution to some problems, the good of the patient being the overwhelming motivating factor. Implicit in this moral obligation to colleagues is the need for maintaining professional competence, for integrity in all her dealings and the use of educated professional judgement at all times.

Because the nurse is the person who provides continuity of care, she is the person closest to the patient and is most likely to gain his confidence and trust. This does not imply that she takes this away from other members of the health team, but rather that she has a unique opportunity, indeed a *moral obligation or duty*, to support and strengthen his confidence and trust in all who minister to him.

Profession

Because the profession of nursing is made up of members of the human race, or fellow men, duty to the profession is included in the section on duty to fellow men. Colleagues, who include nursing colleagues, have just been mentioned as members of the health team. In another dimension the performance or neglect of professional duty by one nurse can affect other practitioners and thus the profession as a whole.

The main points to be remembered here are the following:
- *Maintenance of high standards* of professional practice, which includes keeping up to date – one poor practitioner can damn many good practitioners in the eyes of the public
- *Maintenance of standards of dress and behaviour* which conform with the norms of society and present a good image of the people who practise nursing to the outside world
- *Maintenance of interest in and support for* her professional association, which is part of professionalism
- *Adherence to the accepted code* of nursing ethics in all her professional activities.

Herself

Nurses are human beings, fellow men, and just as they owe a duty to their fellow men so they owe a duty to themselves. Indeed, duty to one's fellow men and to oneself are so interrelated that they are almost inseparable, for one influences the other.

The use of all talents and capabilities to their maximum potential   No two people are alike. This point has been made frequently but is worth repeating, for each person has talents, abilities and capabilities. The human being who chooses nursing as a profession has a moral obligation to develop these faculties to their ultimate potential so as to be able to serve those to whom she has committed herself to the best of her ability. Having chosen nursing as a career means that she must bring a dedication to her studies and practice far greater than that expected of many other categories of workers. The idea of *learning just enough to pass examinations* has no place in nursing, where true education begins with a voyage of discovery towards what is not known and continues throughout the professional life of the nurse. Nothing less is worthy of a practitioner of nursing. It is a duty to herself as well as to her clients/patients.

The pursuit of happiness in the work being done   No person who does not want to do so should become a nurse. Having decided on this career the nurse must seek the sense of achievement inherent in a worthwhile job well done. In reality, the happiness or good of others is what is being sought. The pursuit of happiness is no selfish, egotistical desire – it is only to be found in the realisation of pleasure or the alleviation of suffering that is brought to others by one's acts. It is more than mere personal gratification.

The maintenance of a balanced outlook   This is necessary so that clear thinking can be preserved. This means that an open mind should be cultivated and adequate and varied recreation and interest in life away from the world of work should be pursued so that the needs of fellow-men can be understood and met more adequately.

The maintenance of physical health   This is not simply 'coddling' oneself. Adequate, balanced nutrition and rest and recreation, including exercise, are all part of keeping healthy. It is essential that the nurse who is concerned with caring for the sick should herself be in good health. Her moral obligation to care for herself is obvious.

Meticulous attention to personal appearance and grooming   The nurse who pays attention to her skin, hair and nails and to her general appearance, especially when in uniform, not only adds to her own feeling of well-being but presents a good professional image to her colleagues and patients. Extremes are unnecessary, but it may be necessary to wear one hairstyle when in uniform and another for leisure activities. Patients want nurses to be personable, cheerful but controlled, gentle yet assured in touch and well groomed. In paying attention to herself as regards personal hygiene and grooming, the nurse is performing a service to those for whom she cares.

Maintenance of values and character traits consistent with professional practice and the norms of the society of professional workers of which the nurse is a member. These values include the following:

- *Honesty*, which is an essential quality. Deviations from this may at worst cost a life and at best create unhappiness and lack of trust.

- *Dependability* at all times in serious as well as minor matters. Giving conscientious care to the best of one's ability, whether this is observed or not, is at one end of the scale, but attendance at classes, keeping personal appointments and suchlike matters are equally important.
- *Loyalty* to oneself and to others. This entails self-respect, but with realistic acknowledgement of one's limitations. It also means keeping faith with one's colleagues, refusing to become involved in gossip sessions, and respect for the confidences of patients and others.
- *Readiness to learn* and constant striving to better professional competence and knowledge.
- *Creativity* and the ability to handle emergencies as well as more mundane situations with imagination and resourcefulness and with innovation where necessary.
- *Tolerance*, which enables the nurse to accept others for what they are without prejudice.
- *Discernment*, which includes the exercise of sound professional judgement, leading to the selection of the best course of action in the practice of one's profession and the ability to foresee the consequences of any act performed by oneself or colleagues in the health team so that necessary modifications can be made, for the benefit of clients and/or patients and co-workers.
- *Dignity* and poise in the handling of professional interpersonal relationships.
- *Orderliness*, which includes attention to details such as neatness, methodical performance of tasks and systematic, logical thinking.

All these and more are part of one's duty to oneself and thus to one's fellow men.

The employer

Nurses are very largely employees. The few that are self-employed still owe a duty to the patients or clients who hire their services and the basic principles of their moral obligations to employers also apply to the patient who hires the service of the self-employed nurse.

What does the nurse owe to her employer? It is not very different from what she owes to her patients in general:

- Maintenance of the highest standards of professional competence
- Personal integrity and trustworthiness, her word being her bond
- Maintenance of high ethical standards
- Maintenance of the safety of the patient, his name and property
- Knowledge of and adherence to the philosophy of the employing authority
- Loyalty to the employing authority, physicians and colleagues within the bounds of ethical professional practice
- The courage to question intelligently when things appear to be taking a course which is not considered desirable

- Adherence to rules and regulations, except where these are in direct conflict with the interests of the patient when appropriate measures must be taken to bring any deviations necessary to the attention of those in authority
- Cultivation of good interpersonal relationships with all
- Economic use of supplies and meticulous care of equipment
- Recognition of the fact that the hospital exists for the benefit of the patient and for his care
- Recognition of her responsibilities to the patient, the physician, the employer, her colleagues and her profession.

ATTITUDE OF MIND

In discussing the concept duty it is fitting to touch on the attitude that a nurse brings to her appointed task, for if this is inappropriate then she fails in her duty. A sick person, through no fault of his own, may present a not particularly attractive image. Because she has elected to serve the sick the attitude of the nurse towards the sick person or the person who is worried about his health and fears that he may be or become ill is of tremendous importance. The following may be offered as guidelines for cultivating an appropriate attitude:

- The sick person is a human being and as such is entitled to recognition of his human dignity
- Acceptance of the sick person as he is, a human being in need of care of a specific kind
- Recognition that illness may be even more distasteful to the patient himself than to the nurse or those around him
- Recognition that one of man's most cherished attributes is his independence and that to take this from him, simply because it is 'quicker' or 'easier' to do something oneself, is to negate this attribute
- Avoidance of value judgements about the patient, his culture, background and medical history based on inadequate information. It is all too easy to talk about 'good' patients, 'bad' patients or 'moaners' or to attach the blame of his illness to the patient himself. The nurse must be aware that she may make such value judgements, but because she is aware of this danger she can minimise the effect of such judgements based on her own terms of reference by her attitude towards her patient/client
- Determination always to give of one's best
- A continual quest for knowledge for the betterment of care
- Recognition that others have a right to practise their own religion and to their own opinions
- Thorough knowledge of professional standards of conduct as a basis for all nursing practice
- Care and concern for mankind.

Attitudes do not grow like weeds in a seedbed. They need careful nurturing in the form of training and education and a good teacher, who has as her objective the cultivation of healthy attitudes in her students, will foster observation and the ability to think for themselves in those she is guiding along the road to professional adulthood.

COMPASSION

Compassion is defined as 'pity with, a desire to spare or help'. Compassion seeks to do something about the needs of other people rather than just stand by and feel pity or sorrow – to take active steps to alleviate the cause of the suffering. It also does not mean that the nurse has no feelings for the suffering of patients, that she is indifferent to their distress, but that she is ready and able to do something about it. In order to be able to show compassion she must notice what is happening, observe distress and seek its cause, which may be physical or mental or both, and then marshall action so that treatment is instituted to remove the cause. This treatment will include emotional support where necessary.

Goodwill allied with good intentions does not show compassion unless accompanied by intelligent observation, planning and the implementation of relevant intervention. In other words, by using all the phases of the nursing process allied with the dimension of caring, the nurse is demonstrating compassion of the highest order. The question to ask is 'What is the best thing to do?' and, having found the answer, the nurse must do it. A compassionate person does not sit at a bedside holding a hand unless that is the only way to bring help and comfort, and the emphasis again is on help. Florence Nightingale was compassionate; she saw needs, felt for people in distress, and took very positive, although often unpopular, steps to remedy the wrongs which had led to the unfortunate state of affairs that she found.

Compassion is not a negative but a positive, dynamic state implying deeds rather than words. Compassionate action can lead to the next concept, which is providing a state of well-being.

ACTIVE PROMOTION OF A STATE OF WELL-BEING

Well-being, the state of *being well*, includes mental as well as physical 'being well'. It is this idea that underlies all good therapy, of whatever sort and in whatever circumstances, that the health care team strives to provide. Again the *active* nature of this function is important.

Complete well-being may not be attainable, but relative well-being is always possible. In endeavours to promote the former it is quite possible that the latter may be achieved. Even when severely ill, the patient, who is made and kept comfortable, free from pain, and with a mind at ease is in a state of relative well-being which has been attained through team-work, thoughtful, intelligent care and positive action. In nursing, the active promotion of well-being consists of giving to others, often also in collaboration with others, that for which one's skill and training equips one. The means for achieving physical and mental well-being vary with the circumstances and each member of the health team and the patient and his family have to make their own contribution towards its attainment.

In the context of duty, the *active* promotion of well-being, physical and mental, complete or relative, is a function that a nurse ought to undertake. It is something that she should, indeed *must*, do.

CONFLICT OF DUTY

While it is often easy to determine what should be done, that is where one's duty lies, in medicine there are many grey areas where duties conflict and a decision may be extremely difficult to make. This can be a very practical problem and can cause much soul-searching in the medical and nursing profession where common generalisations, which attempt to formulate norms that are valid for all can, in special circumstances, lead to difficulties and conflicts. These generalisations include, *inter alia*, the following:

☐ Serve God before man.
☐ One's duty to one's family comes before that to strangers.
☐ Follow your conscience and you can't go wrong.
☐ Put others before yourself.
☐ Save life at all costs.

Solutions to problems are not offered – there are too many variables involved, but a few examples will serve to illustrate how conflicts can arise.

Serve God before man In the first instance it might occur that a doctor or nurse receives a call to emergency work which, if obeyed, would prevent attendance at church. Of course the doctor or nurse would not hesitate to answer the call to emergency work. In fact, to the religious, this may be regarded as a service to God. However, frequent routine work-shifts which seriously interfere with attendance at church could cause conflict for the nurse when she may see routine work, which other staff members appear to be escaping from as conflicting with her duty regarding religious observance. This may seem to be a situation that is not too difficult to overcome, but is it, in practice, always so?

One's duty towards one's family may often conflict with one's duty to *strangers*, who in this case are clients or patients. Does it follow that the dictum quoted above always applies? The nurse's code of ethics makes her patient of paramount importance, but a nursing sister who has a sick child may find the commonly held norm that the family comes first to conflict with the ethical norm that the patient comes first and have understandable difficulty in resolving this problem.

Follow your conscience and you can't go wrong is also an over-simplification, for one person's conscience may lead her to a decision that one action is right while another equally 'mature' person may come to a completely opposite conclusion about the right action to take in the same set of circumstances.

Who is 'right'? Both points of view may appear to be quite logical. The best solution may be to agree to differ, but someone must make the decision to act. This responsibility will rest with the team leader in the health care system. The rest of the team may have to carry out that decision even if it goes against their consciences. 'They can withdraw', you say? Again this is an over-simplification. Is the patient then left without attention because of that withdrawal? Of course the nurse who knows that the hospital policy conflicts with the dictates of her conscience should not work there, but this does not justify her staging a walk-out which would leave patients with no care. That is also morally indefensible.

Put others before yourself also sounds simple in the nursing context, but is it really? For how long do you put others before yourself? – until you drop from exhaustion or your health suffers? In the long run are you not of less use to others with your efficiency impaired by fatigue or ill-health? It has already been stated that nurses have a duty to themselves in order to fulfil their duty or obligations to others. Moderation in all things would seem to be a guide to solving a problem of this nature.

Save life at all costs is easy to say and difficult to carry out. *Whose* life, when many are involved – the life of a patient suffering from terminal cancer who has a cardiac arrest? Many similar examples could be quoted. There is no easy answer. Where does one's duty or moral obligations lie – certainly not in actively promoting death, but in passively allowing it to occur? This can be a very traumatic conflict situation tied up with questions concerning the sanctity of life.

These and many other examples could be quoted. In pointing out that there may be conflicts about what is considered to be duty, it is hoped that understanding may be brought to many situations in the nursing field where seeming conflicts of duty occur.

8 Accountability

Accountability is a term that is bandied about today. Often it is feared, with little understanding of its meaning and implications. The word 'accountable' is defined as 'bound to give account' or 'responsible' (*Concise Oxford Dictionary*, 4th ed), while an 'account' is a 'reckoning of debit or credit in money or service' or a 'report'. Today society demands that account be given not only of money spent (usually public money), but also of service rendered by people giving that service, people who are often in the employ of the state.

Professional people, irrespective of whether they are paid by the state, must also be held accountable for their acts and omissions. The control of professional behaviour, of ethical conduct, is vested in the profession itself. Nurses are subject to disciplinary control by their statutory governing body, which is the South African Nursing Council in South Africa. This body lays down broad ethical codes and ensures that those who violate these or are accused of so doing are subjected to inquiry and trial by their peers.

If nurses are accountable for their actions, if they have to show justification for what they do, then there should be some clarification regarding *who* is accountable in nursing, *to whom* and *for what*. The ethical code of behaviour underlying the profession of nursing has already received attention, as has the concept duty in the nursing context. The nurse is, in the framework of this chapter, the one who is accountable. She is, as a professional person, required to assume responsibility for her acts and omissions in the performance of her professional tasks and is bound to give account, or 'make a report', or 'give reckoning' of service for her professional actions. The nurse is the *who* in this context, but *to whom* is she accountable and *for what*?

TO WHOM IS THE NURSE ACCOUNTABLE?

In many cases this can be answered by looking at those to whom the nurse owes a moral responsibility or duty as spelt out in the preceding chapter, but because accountability has a more specific connotation, requiring as it does the giving of an account of service, it is approached from a different angle. Thus those to whom the nurse is accountable include the following:

The client or patient

The client or patient depends on the faithful service of the nurse and entrusts himself or a member of his family to her care. In many cases he also foots the bill, either by means of direct payment for services rendered or indirectly by taxation. It seems something of a paradox that the payers of the highest taxes are sometimes denied access to treatment at the institutions their taxes help to maintain. The nurse is thus doubly accountable for service to the individual as a person in need of care and as a taxpayer.

The employer

This can be an individual or an employing authority. In the vast majority of cases nurses are employed by bodies such as provincial administrations or municipalities. These bodies are maintained by public monies and have to account for their expenditure of monies on services. The salaries of nurses comprise at least 60% of all the monies expended on health services. There is no doubt that a nurse can be held accountable for her service by those who employ her.

The medical practitioner

Although the nurse has many independent functions, she is nevertheless charged with the care of clients or patients who are also the clients or patients of the medical practitioner, and thus has a dual accountability.

Her colleagues and her profession

The nurse is accountable to her nursing colleagues and thus to her profession, for she forms part of the whole and cannot escape from this responsibility while she practises her profession. What she does and how she carries out her professional tasks reflects on the profession as a whole.

The public

Who are the potential clients or patients for whom she will care? John Citizen, who contributes a large amount through taxation and donation to the establishment and maintenance of the health service and to the education of those practising the various professions that keep these services operating. Nursing is one of these professions. The professional nurse also forms part of the health team responsible for assessing the health care needs in the community and the way these are met. She is also a member of that public to whom she is accountable.

The students of the profession

Although the neophyte nurse is a member of the profession, she is so important that she merits a section to herself, for many registered nurses fail to realise that they are accountable to the students of today who are the registered nurses of the future. The guidance given to the student to assist her in achieving her role as a useful professional adult is of the utmost importance to her development and is part of the concept accountability in nursing.

The type of service will vary in the different fields of nursing, but basic principles remain the same.

FOR WHAT IS THE NURSE ACCOUNTABLE?

Having identified some of the people or categories of people to whom the nurse is accountable, we will now look at them separately and clarify the specific accountability of the nurse in each area.

The client or patient

The nurse is accountable for, *inter alia*, the following:

- [ ] Maintaining professional competence so that quality care is always given
- [ ] Keeping her knowledge up to date
- [ ] Observing and reporting on the condition and progress of those in her care
- [ ] Accurate record-keeping
- [ ] Maintenance of the safety of the person's name, person and property
- [ ] Evaluating the quality of care given by herself and those working with her, so that improvement in the quality of care remains constantly before all as the ultimate goal. Nothing is ever perfect, but nurses must strive to make the quality of care as near perfect as possible
- [ ] Supervising the environment in which care is given and those giving that nursing care
- [ ] Maintaining her own health so that she may function optimally in her nursing service
- [ ] Helping the client/patient to utilise whatever potential he has to maintain optimal health.

The employer

Again the nurse has special areas where her accountability is clear. These include the following:

- [ ] Maintaining professional competence and knowledge
- [ ] Managing a department or unit entrusted to her care
- [ ] Economic use and safe keeping of equipment and supplies provided for her to render care. This includes pharmaceutical supplies and drugs, food, medical supplies and equipment, linen, etc. The able management of personnel also falls into this category
- [ ] Observing and reporting unfavourable conditions in the environment, in the equipment or supplies and unsatisfactory performance on the part of personnel
- [ ] Accurate reporting
- [ ] Employing all measures necessary to prevent or minimise medico-legal hazards

- Rendering a full day's work for a full day's pay and ensuring that other personnel do the same
- Cooperating with other members of the health team for quality patient care
- Knowledge of policy and the implementation thereof, except where this is in direct conflict with the interest of the patients or ethical codes. In this case the difficulties must be reported and discussed so that solutions can be found
- Use of the correct channels of communication to ensure the smooth running of the organisation
- Leadership and guidance to the less experienced members of the nursing team
- Maintaining her own health and caring for those working in her team.

The medical practitioner
The following points are especially relevant:

- In carrying out prescribed treatment for the medical officer's patient/client, it must always be remembered that the nurse is responsible for her own acts and omissions so that, although the doctor prescribes treatment, the nurse is herself responsible or accountable for the manner in which she carries it out
- Observing a patient's progress, including progress or regression, and reaction to medication in other forms of treatment
- Accurate reporting and recording
- Emergency action where necessary
- Maintaining professional competence
- Participating in research
- Use of intelligent judgement.

Her colleagues and her profession
- Maintaining the highest ethical standards
- Maintaining professional competence
- Maintaining a professional image
- Participating in activities which will promote the interests of the profession.

The public
- Maintaining professional competence
- Maintaining ethical standards
- Constant vigilance for possible health hazards
- Confidentiality
- Research to find methods of improving nursing care and to determine needs

- [ ] Health education
- [ ] Proper use of resources provided.

The student

In this respect there is a two-fold responsibility or two areas where accountability has particular significance.

Clinical area Nurses are 'doers', but their doing is related to knowing *what to do, how to do, when to do, where to do* and, most important of all, *why to do*. Their work is related to the clinical area of nursing in some way or other, for even the nurse administrator, who sometimes seems far from the side of the patient or client receiving clinical care, is responsible for facilitating care. If the nurse has to *do* and know what, how, when, where and why *to do*, it follows that she must be taught and guided to professional competence and judgement. The persons most intimately concerned with this teaching and guidance are those with whom she comes into contact most often, namely registered nurses in the clinical area. These vital members of the health care team are accountable to the neophytes and students for the following:

- [ ] Constant guidance and assistance along the road to professional adulthood. A registered nurse in the clinical situation, being responsible for patient care, must teach her students how to give that care or she fails in her accountability to the patient/client for whose care she is answerable. She must therefore teach the students, or pupils, or other members of her team. It is an inescapable part of her task. In the present pattern of staff allocation students and pupils form part of the team. However, they are not there as a pair of hands, but as learners of nursing practice
- [ ] Maintenance of their own standards of professional competence, knowledge and ethical standards so that they form a good role model for the students, pupils and others
- [ ] Ensuring that they, the registered nurses, are aware of the educational needs of students and pupils and that they strive at all times to meet these needs. Nurses are members of the general student body and should be well aware of the type of education they are receiving and of the accountability of clinical educators, who are the registered nurses working in the ward situation.

Formal teaching area Unfortunately, a division has grown up between clinical practice, or the so-called 'service' area, and the 'formal teaching' college or lecture room area. There are many good practical reasons for this which it is not necessary to consider here. While this dichotomy exists, and while it is still impractical for nurse educators to move more completely into the clinical scene, those concerned with the formal teaching area of nursing education are accountable to their students for the following:

- [ ] Relevance of what is taught
- [ ] Up-to-date knowledge
- [ ] Thoughtful curriculum planning

- ☐ Carefully chosen presentation
- ☐ Objective evaluation
- ☐ Constant guidance
- ☐ Provision of an environment conducive to learning, including educational facilities such as books, models, tapes, films, etc
- ☐ Seeing the students or pupils as their *raison d'etre* – in other words, if there were no students or pupils there would be no need for nurse educators
- ☐ Maintenance of high ethical standards.

In both areas the neophyte is being prepared to meet the nursing component of health care needs for quality care. The teachers in both areas are accountable to their students for providing *quality nursing education* so that the student may be led to recognition of personal accountability in her professional life, so that decision making with regard to patient care can be based on soundly developed professional judgement acquired by correlation of theory and practice into one indivisible whole.

GENERAL COMMENTS

The concept accountability is not new, but in the practical application it has changed. Where once it was a desirable value to obey the orders of superiors without question this is no longer the case. The old expression 'Theirs not to question why, theirs but to do or die' has no place in the world today. Unquestioning obedience to the order of another, without thought or regard for the effect of an action on others, is condemned.

The long-established influence of religious training and of the military nursing orders on the development of nursing tended to enshrine the role model of the nurse carrying out instructions given by someone higher up in the medical or nursing hierarchy as a duty. The superior 'officer' was held responsible for the consequences of the actions of the 'inferior'. This has changed. The excuse 'I was just carrying out orders' is no longer accepted as valid.

Sweeping changes have occurred in religious orders – personal accountability in matters of conscience, 'thinking for oneself' is accepted – and in military matters, where officers have been held personally responsible for the killing of innocent civilians despite the plea that they were 'carrying out orders'. The results of 'carrying out these orders' were obvious to those executing the orders, and they could have refrained or stopped the action which led to casualties. The concept of personal accountability was accepted by military authorities and society in general, and the personal culpability of the perpetrators was established. One such case in point, which received wide publicity, was the 'My Lai' incident in the Vietnamese war.

The relevance for nursing is that the nursing hierarchy and pattern of organisation is built largely on the religious sisterhoods and the military pattern. Both have profoundly influenced nursing practice. If personal accountability is accepted in these two fields of endeavour, then surely nursing must not lag behind.

In the education of the modern nurse the emphasis is on producing an educated, thinking being, capable of observation, nursing diagnosis and action. She is trained to use the nursing process to assess the situation and to evolve a plan, short-term or long-term as the need arises, including emergency action. She carries out the plan herself or ensures that it is implemented in a team effort. She evaluates the effect of action, good or bad, and records the actions and the results, reassesses the situation, re-plans, re-implements, re-evaluates and continues to record for so long as she is responsible or accountable for that patient/client/person's care.

Omission is as serious as commission. Accountability means that culpability is assigned to anyone neglecting to perform the service for which he or she has been prepared. 'I did not notice' and 'Nobody told me' are not ways of fulfilling the obligation to give account for service rendered or, in this case, not rendered.

Automation and technology in modern developed societies are reducing the job opportunities available to those without training. They have also made the types of skills and practices required of the professional more and more complex. The education of the professional nurse is, with very few exceptions, paid for by the taxpayer. Modern medical and nursing knowledge has reduced the length of the patient's stay in hospital. At the same time it has increased the cost of treatment and hospitalisation. A factor that is often overlooked is that because of the efficiency of treatment, which is thus of shorter duration, the cost per illness has remained much the same. The nurse, who is generally educated by the state, is accountable for using that education to give quality care and to minimise hazards inherent in the health care system so that the cost per illness is kept as low as possible. Her acts or omissions must always show that she understands her personal accountability and that this underlies all her professional practice.

Another aspect that perhaps bears brief examination is the question of the 'good nurse' and the 'good patient'. The 'good' nurse has not gone, but her role has evolved with the cultural and social changes that have occurred. She works a 40-hour week and earns a reasonable salary. The *good old* nurse' probably worked six 12-hour shifts and earned very little. Her education was more on-the-job. She was thus 'seen' by patients; 72 hours per week meant that every patient was likely to see that nurse for a considerable period during the six days with one day off-duty per week.

The nurse of today may work as follows:

Monday	07h00 – 15h00
Tuesday	Off
Wednesday	Off
Thursday	14h00 – 22h00
Friday	14h00 – 22h00
Saturday	07h00 – 15h00
Sunday	07h00 – 15h00

If a patient is admitted to hospital at 16h00 on Monday and is discharged at 10h00 on Friday, he may have encountered that particular nurse for eight hours on Thursday, during which time he may have slept for at least two hours, and have been discharged on Friday before she came on duty. Other nurses who may have cared for him on Tuesday might have been off-duty on Wednesday and Thursday, so that the continuity of contact with nurses may have been impossible. This does not mean that the quality of care would have been inferior, nor that the accountability of those giving that care would have been less than in the 'good old days'. It may easily have been more, for the treatment and possible side-effects could have been much more. Social as well as medical care changes have, in effect, increased the accountability of those rendering the care.

The concept of the *'good submissive patient'* has also changed as a result of social change. He is better educated and better informed about his illness and his financial contribution to the cost, direct or indirect, is usually high. Radio, television, books and magazines and even advertisements make him much more questioning about his treatment and his progress. After all, 'he' is being treated. The progress is 'his' progress. Is he not entitled to know what is happening to him?

Modern medical practice advocates the inclusion of the patient in the planning and carrying out of his own treatment. Passive submission is regarded as a sign that there is something seriously wrong with him; active participation is considered vital. Are today's nurses really geared to meet these changes? They are being educated along these lines, but do they see this as part of their accountability? Do they see themselves as bound to give account, responsible for this encouragement of patient participation and responsible for explaining why it is necessary for them to 'do this', 'take that' or 'avoid this', or do they still make use of the easy way out: *'because the doctor says so'*? Keeping patients in helpless ignorance is outdated.

In concluding this section on accountability it is suggested that nurses should take a long, hard look at themselves and their professional practice so that they are fully aware of what accountability embraces in their work and are ready and able at all times and in all places to give account of the service which, because of their professional commitment, they are bound to render to their patients or clients, to the members of the health team, to those who employ them, to their colleagues and to their profession. In so doing they will uphold the proud tradition of the past and build a solid foundation for the future.

9 Discipline in the nursing context

Discipline related to nursing or nurses is mentioned so frequently in literature that a work on the ethos of nursing cannot omit at least a brief look at this concept. The word is derived from the Latin *disciplina* from *discipulus* (disciple), and may mean a 'branch of instruction' hence the discipline of medicine, or of nursing or of sociology, etc. It may be a 'trained condition', a 'system of rules for conduct or control exercised over', and the verb means to 'bring under control, train to obedience and order'.

Thus discipline in nursing can be the subject of nursing science itself, the trained condition of the nurse who follows a system of rules for professional conduct, can apply to the control exercised over professional practice and can refer to the orderly functioning of the profession of nursing. It is proposed to examine each of these aspects separately from the point of view of what the discipline entails, who applies it and how, and whether it is internal (self-discipline) or external (imposed from outside), or whether both internal and external discipline play a part.

THE DISCIPLINE OF NURSING

This means, in effect, the branch of instruction or study that is followed, namely the *art and science of nursing*.

Nursing has already been defined in the first chapter. The instruction or study necessary for one who is to follow the profession of nursing is long and varied, based on the sciences and the humanities and uses related disciplines freely in order to build its own body of knowledge. The art and science of nursing is a unique, dynamic discipline with a body of professional practitioners requiring a great deal of educated, specialised judgement, coupled with practised technical skill which is based on knowledge derived from the natural and biological sciences, as well as on the social sciences. This knowledge is used to enable the nursing process with its elements of assessment of nursing needs, planning nursing action, implementation of the nursing plan and evaluation of the results of action together with the necessary recording, to be carried out for the benefit of the patient or client being served, within the framework of the independent, interdependent and dependent functions of the nurse, her ethical code and with due regard to her accountability. In this she must become a master of her art and science. The nurse's unique function is complex, including the giving of physical care, carrying out her part of the total therapeutic plan and giving emotional support to the patient/client and to the wider circle of his family and friends while at all times assisting other members of the health team and coordinating their activities. Thus the discipline of nursing covers a very wide field indeed.

The discipline of nursing is practised by the practitioners of nursing. They, by means of their peer-group control, determine the field of study, that is they lay down syllabuses for the training of neophytes. They make rules and regulations to ensure that the education of the professional, semi-professional and also the nurse's assistant complies with minimum standards. They conduct examinations which lead to certification of competency and to registration or enrolment. They prescribe the mechanism for registration or enrolment and its maintenance. They provide for post-basic training programmes as these are needed and they control these programmes. Through their professional association they encourage, if not actively promote, the education of nurses at all levels to ensure high standards of professional education. They are instrumental in getting new and better educational facilities for nurses of all categories. They write professional literature, they undertake nursing research. Nurses are active in promoting the discipline of nursing and in furthering its aims.

Discipline as control

In the sense of *having control over* or *bringing under control* nursing is mainly affected because it is concerned with activities which affect the well-being and even the lives of other human beings. Nursing, too, as part of its armentarium uses medications, techniques and equipment that have high risk potentials. Nurses are also servants of the public, financed largely by public monies.

It follows that the practice of nursing has to have controls, some of which are imposed from outside by means of the laws of the land (here drug control is an easily understood example), by means of state, provincial, municipal or local employing authorities. It also requires a measure of control by the profession itself and by members of the profession as individuals.

Controls are not established for the sake of applying petty tyranny and *making life difficult*. They are there for the protection of the client or patient who may, at some stage of his progress through the health care system, be in a very dependent state. They also exist for the protection of the employing authorities. It must never be forgotten that controls also exist to protect the nurse.

The authority of those exercising control is conferred in various ways. The right to require or demand certain actions from other people in the nursing world may be derived from the following:

Appointment The role and status of a person appointed to a particular post gives that person the authority to exercise discipline over or control the action of others. Thus the nursing service manager controls the sister, the sister the student, the medical superintendent other medical practitioners on the staff, and the chief administrator the clerical staff in a hospital. These are very simple examples to illustrate the point. No doubt many more will spring to mind. This appointment to authority to control should be accompanied by an adequate job description of the role to be filled, with clearly delineated lines of authority.

Election The person in whom authority is vested is elected formally for a specific purpose for a given period. The president of a professional association is elected by the group. The first step is usually election of members of the profession to the governing body and then the smaller group elects one of its members to the office of president, with its attendant responsibilities and powers which include control over others.

Common consent This type of authority or control mechanism is much more informal. One member of a group takes charge of nursing actions because of her superior skills in and knowledge of a particular situation. This is a much more fluid form of control which changes as different needs arise. It is often the type of leadership that emerges in an emergency situation and falls away once the crisis is passed.

Seized This is a form of dictatorship where authority over others is taken and held by force. It has no place in nursing.

Supervision as discipline and control

Supervision, that is 'directing or watching with authority the work or proceedings or progress of,' is well-known in nursing. It is, of course, a control measure, a means of keeping order, but it entails more than simply standing and watching, even with authority, for it has as its object the assurance that quality care is given. If this is true then correction and teaching form a very large part of supervision in nursing. Supervision does not entail playing policeman.

Nursing, like any other form of activity that involves some form of action, is undertaken to attain an objective. Quality nursing care is the basic objective of nursing. This is a difficult concept, for it must be determined exactly what the quality care for which nursing is striving is. It is for this reason that supervision of care is undertaken. The person upon whom the task of ensuring quality care falls, must have criteria against which she can measure the nursing action. These criteria are established either by joint decision or consensus or by the knowledge and experience gained by the practitioner. The supervisor herself must be a competent practitioner who is constantly on the look-out for new and improved methods of performance and who is prepared to share these with others and help them to attain greater proficiency.

The overall purpose of control by supervision is to compare actual performance with that which was envisaged. Through supervision it should be possible to determine not only whether all those entitled to receive health care do actually receive it, but also whether the services rendered are performed by those competent to do so in an approved manner. If there are deficiencies then it is up to the supervisor to ensure that these deficiencies are remedied by teaching, rearrangement of personnel and task assignment and the provision of physical facilities at least sufficient to meet needs. Failure to do so constitutes negligence. The supervisor of nursing is not there to report, reprimand and punish, but to observe, praise where praise is due and remedy where necessary. The supervisor who throws her weight and authority around is not fulfilling her function.

The supervisor of nursing is responsible, or accountable, for the overall nursing care and service function of the nursing personnel assigned to her charge. She plays a part in assessing the needs of patients/clients for nursing care, assigning nursing personnel to carry out the care and evaluating the quality of the care given. She directs, assists, trains, educates and instructs nursing personnel regarding nursing practice, including the provision of a safe environment in which safe, efficient therapy can be offered. The maintenance of morale by helping those who are unsure of their techniques or competence, or who need guidance in their interpersonal relationships with patients/clients, colleagues and other members of the health team, is part of the whole picture.

Supervision starts early in nursing. The neophyte is often supervised by members of her peer group, themselves students, who have already attained a measure of nursing care skills. If this situation is properly appreciated and handled as a teaching-learning situation, then the assumption of more and more responsibility for supervision in the work situation develops naturally, so that the future supervisor of complex nursing care learns and practises skills as she travels the road to full professional maturity.

One of the most important members of the supervision team is the clinical teacher, who in her task of ensuring that the student acquires mastery over the principles of professional practice and by increasing her competence at all levels has a supervisory function. Unless the clinical teacher observes what the student is doing, in other words unless she 'watches with authority', and unless she assesses, evaluates and guides, she is not fulfilling one of her most fundamental tasks. A clear concept of what the student must *know* in order to be able *to do* is as necessary as clarity on what constitutes '*good doing*'.

Inspection

Whether on a small scale by a departmental head, or on a large scale by the Director of Nursing Services, inspection is a more remote form of supervision. Its aim and objective is the same, namely to ensure that what should be done is being done, by capable people, in the best manner possible, at the proper time, for the correct reason and with due regard to safety of the recipient's person, his name and his property. It may entail the use of detailed checklists, or may be more informal. It is a control measure, and as such is a means of applying discipline. It is a common measure for applying control and should never degenerate into negative fault-finding and criticism. Advice on remedial measures to be taken is of more value than a detailed report spelling out faults. It should be positive in what it does.

Discipline and breaches of discipline

It has already been pointed out that control measures entail the use of rules and regulations. There must also, therefore, be some form of penalty applied when these are broken. Rules and regulations for the control of professional practice exist to safeguard the public, which is the recipient of care, the authorities, which run the service, and the members of the health team, including the nurses, who supply the service.

The nurse is subject, through her registering body, to disciplinary control for conduct that can be considered improper or disgraceful with regard to her profession. Mechanisms exist for investigating alleged misconduct, for peer-group trial of accused members of the profession, and for the application of various forms of sanction against those found guilty. These sanctions can take the form of removal from the register or roll, suspension, reprimand and cautioning or, in the case of students, prolongation of the period of training. This procedure is in line with that followed by other professions. Thus if the offence is sufficiently serious, discipline used in this sense may make it impossible for the guilty person to carry on practising his profession. Other offences, considered to be less serious, have lesser penalties.

In nursing practice it is often necessary for a member of the profession to judge those lower in the hierarchy for alleged *breaches of discipline*. The following guidelines might be of relevance for such nurses.

Investigate the incident fully from all angles to determine:
- [ ] the exact nature of the offence
- [ ] whether the rule or regulation was known to the offender, and if not, why not
- [ ] the consequences of the offence, either actual or potential
- [ ] the mechanisms for using adequate safeguards
- [ ] whether the offence was committed for the first time or whether it was of a persistent nature (the person who comes on duty late once may have a very good reason for it; persistent lateness requires not only investigation, but action)
- [ ] any mitigating circumstances.

Having investigated, take appropriate action This may entail the application of punishment or sanctions, it might equally well entail the application of better methods of control, remedying untenable situations or specific education or re-education.

Re-check to see that the situation does not occur again, both in the short and in the long term.

If the application of sanctions and discipline in this context is part of the functional activity of particular staff members, then this should be spelt out in their job descriptions and clearly understood by all concerned, both up and down the hierarchy pertaining to that service. The method of maintaining discipline may be formal or informal, but where subordinates fail to observe the prescribed standards of conduct with regard to their duties it may be necessary to subject them to formal disciplinary measures. Proper authority to do so must be vested in those entrusted with the enforcement of these penalties.

Discipline and external control

So far all the measures discussed have been those of imposed discipline, discipline or control that comes from outside. All hospital and health services are governed by external control which includes Acts of Parliament, provincial ordinances and municipal by-laws. Legislative bodies have laid down rules and regulations which must be complied with when health services are supplied.

In order to ensure compliance written reports are usually required, at least on an annual basis. These incorporate statistics which show how the budget has been spent to supply these services and the results obtained. Questions can be asked in meetings of legislative bodies, select committees can be appointed and the auditing of accounts is provided for. Courts of law are there to deal with malpractice. Delegated power must be open to examination. External control or discipline *is* necessary, but it must also be subject to scrutiny so that rules and regulations are examined periodically to see whether they still apply.

Self-discipline or internal discipline

This is perhaps one of the most difficult aspects to be considered. On its own it could take up a whole book, or at least a chapter, but it will be touched upon very briefly in the context of the nurse and nursing.

Self-discipline or internal discipline comes from the individual himself. It is internal to him and not imposed from outside. It is part of cultural background and a way of life. It governs the actions of the individual and his pattern of behaviour. He learns it as part of the socialisation process. If it is so individual, what does it have to do with nursing? This can be answered quite simply by pointing out that although the nurse is an individual, the very nature of her profession – which is dedicated to the care of others – makes it necessary that she controls her actions and emotions so that her deeds never cause harm or hurt to those entrusted to her ministrations (it must be remembered that 'to minister to' means 'to serve').

Self-discipline is part of the lifestyle of mature adults. It must be even more so that of mature professional adults. The professional nurse has to discipline herself to observe, to study and to combine knowledge and observation to apply the nursing process. Others can teach, can show the way, but they cannot observe or learn for you. They cannot draw conclusions for you. In order to function as a professional person from whom educated judgements in the practice of your profession are expected, you, and only you, can exercise control.

The curriculum may be imposed. Making its contents your own requires you to control yourself and your actions, that is to apply self-discipline so that you direct yourself to the mastery of subject matter and combine it with what you already know for your own benefit and that of others.

The concept self-discipline is often interpreted in the narrow sense of not allowing yourself to do things, of controlling emotions and generally restricting your own freedom of action, if not of thought. True self-discipline, because it allows you to exercise control over your actions, your plans and your observations, frees your mind to think as objectively as possible and to apply the results of such thought and judgement to the benefit of those you serve. What comes from within is part of you, for your own decisions made it possible. In the long term self-control to a large extent does away with external control, or makes it a pleasurable experience, for you are able to measure up to all the demands of external control. External control, which is designed to safeguard the interests of the recipients of nursing care and those who supply it, is easily understood and accepted by those who practise considered self-control.

Acceptance of authority

Although it has been said that the person who exercises reasoned self-control in the practice of her profession accepts control and thus order or discipline, the attitude of mind and emotions of those who are placed in authority and who have to maintain control also require some attention.

Control, discipline, authority – call it what you will – is necessary to maintain the smooth running of services. It is not always easy for those made responsible for ensuring that health services function properly to accept the authority vested in them. Basically a nurse becomes a nurse to help and serve people. She sees this as an individual contract between herself and those she serves and other members of the health team. Soon, however, she finds that she does not do everything for one person. Functional nursing, which is very task orientated, or distributive nursing, which entails performing certain nursing acts for people who need them outside the health service supply agency, while other services are performed by the patients, their families or friends, makes for fragmentation of care. The higher up the hierarchy the student progresses, the more the skilled techniques fall to her lot until one day she becomes a registered nurse. If she remains in the hospital care system she then starts to move away from the bed or patient's side to a managerial role, and her nursing skills are used more in the exercise of judgement and the planning of nursing care than in the actual supply thereof.

Unless she becomes a private-day nurse or 'specials' a patient, she does not give total patient care although she may ensure that it is given. Usually the progression to the exercising of authority is a gradual and painless one, but there are many young, inexperienced registered nurses who find themselves with responsibility and authority that they do not want or are afraid to exercise. Is this not one of the reasons why some 'sisters' shy away from teaching in the ward and from too much patient contact by becoming so bogged down with *administrative* tasks that they are *too busy* to attend to their teaching functions? Nurses would do well to reflect on this. Imposing authority upon others may be very difficult for some people.

If rules and regulations are absolutely necessary to the functioning of a service and the reasons behind them are understood they are usually acceptable to those under that authority, but there may be rebels who do not conform. Authoritarian 'do as I tell you' methods seldom produce lasting results. Reasoned argument and discussion, with a full explanation of the need for the rule and justification of its imposition, will achieve more. The basic aim of all rules, regulations and the imposition of authority must be to ensure the well-being of patients/clients and colleagues and the smooth functioning of the organisation as a whole so that well-being can be achieved and maintained.

Nursing as a *branch of instruction* is a *discipline* followed by persons who are *trained* for it and who adhere to a *system of rules of conduct* in order to render a service to people. It is of necessity an *ordered* profession, dealing as it does with the lives and well-being of others. Discipline entails authority, both the exercising thereof and the acceptance of necessary control. Self-discipline is vital to the practitioners of the discipline of nursing.

10 Some other aspects of nursing

If nursing has as its objective the rendering of quality care to those human beings in need of a special type of care, then it is necessary that a study of the ethos of nursing concerns itself with not only the historical trends throughout the development of nursing from early times until the present day, but also the evolution of various methods to facilitate the provision of that care. Two of the most important aspects will receive attention, namely nursing administration and nursing education. Both are essential if nursing care is to be efficient, effective and socially acceptable to the recipients, to those who give the care and to those who finance its provision.

The type of care given to the sick depends to a large extent on the level of culture of the people on the receiving end and the way these people think. It is very closely linked with the intellectual development, economic status and social conditions existing in the community served. Scientific and technological progress also acts as a determinant.

The modern concept of comprehensive care, which is orientated towards promotive and preventive rather than curative work, has not reached all members of society, nor has a total acceptance of society's responsibility for health care been achieved. As the extent of health care increased the manner in which it was provided became more organised. Nursing administration as we understand it today had its origins in this organisational pattern.

NURSING ADMINISTRATION

The meaning of the concept nurse has changed from an attendant of good behaviour and clean habits, kind and skilled in giving service to patients (including cooking food, rubbing the limbs, lifting the patient or assisting him to walk, making beds, washing patients, waiting upon those who were ailing and willingly carrying out orders of a physician), to a highly trained professional person who forms an essential part of the health team. Today's nurse requires more than common sense, kindness and sympathy.

The modern nurse has to be capable of applying management principles so as to ensure care for her patients. Hospitals existed in ancient Greece, Rome, Egypt and India during the pre-Christian period. Ancient writings, including those of Charaka and Susruta in India, discuss matters such as hospital facilities and the duties of nurses or attendants.

The hospital is and always has been a social organisation that has grown up to meet specific social needs. It has varied in complexity from being simply a place where the sick were housed to the highly complex organisation that it is today. During the early Christian period 'ministering' to a patient was regarded as a way of atoning for sins. Hospitals proliferated, being set up as hospices for travellers and those overcome by disaster.

During the Middle Ages hospitals were dirty, dark, miserable, damp buildings overrun by pests. They were places where the aged, the orphaned and the poor were housed. It was only during the fourteenth century that the attention of those responsible for hospitals shifted to the treatment of the sick and injured. The objective of protecting health by admitting those infected with what were thought to be dangerous diseases also came to the fore. During the Reformation hospital care was unbelievably bad, except in some religiously controlled hospitals. The administration of hospitals was extremely poor; nursing administration was non-existent.

With the Renaissance things began to improve. Voluntary hospitals were organised. They were financed and controlled by wealthy citizens. Some were controlled by church organisations, others by lay people. All were influenced by the effects of industrialism and capitalism, which produced wealthy tycoons as well as more ill-health, and by the general changes in thought brought about by the study of the humanities and an awakening of the public conscience. Gradually the concept of health care provision and state responsibility for hospitals became a reality.

Hospitals became not only places where medical practice was applied to the treatment of patients and the latest developments of science and technology were available (which in themselves demanded organisation and management skills), but also places where medical men received training and experience. In the wake of this development of hospitals and medicine the need for nurses who were better prepared for the roles that were evolving, for the practice of professional nursing which was properly organised and controlled, arose. Training or education to meet these needs became essential.

Nursing personnel in the hospitals of the nineteenth and early twentieth centuries were expected to be motivated by the dedication to service which originated in the Middle Ages. They worked long hours, performing many tasks that were purely domestic in nature. Medical care was expanding and nursing practice was also expanding to keep pace with new needs. The nurse required more education, more 'training', but service needs often took precedence so that training was relegated to the nurses' free time. Exploitation was rife. Authoritarianism and paternalism characterised what nursing administration there was. Medical men developed a great measure of autonomy of action, even when their patients were treated in state or semi-state hospitals. Nurses and nursing lagged behind.

Because patients have to be nursed 24 hours a day, many nurses were needed in hospitals and in other services providing health care. Because the matron (or director of nursing) functioned in an autocratic setting, she established a power structure in which her word was law. As services expanded and nursing service began to be seen as a separate entity in the hospital milieu a definite management structure responsible for the administration of nursing services in collaboration with those of other departments had to be created.

Florence Nightingale played her part in proving the worth of good nursing. Health programmes expanded and more nurses were needed to care for more patients. However, their professional and economic status left much to be desired. Change was in the air. Studies of nursing functions, nursing practice and nursing care were conducted. Various methods of providing patient care were studied and analysed. Nurse leaders and nurse educators emerged who were active in helping to devise ways of ensuring the provision of nursing care that was not only adequate but of a high quality.

Adequate staffing standards were investigated and continue to undergo scrutiny as new patient care needs emerge. New techniques, equipment, instruments and medications abound in nursing practice. The electronic age has produced computerised patient records and even diagnosis. It has been stated that 90% of all medications used by modern physicians today did not exist even ten years ago. Diagnostic techniques become more sophisticated by the day, if not by the hour. Socio-economic conditions, a citizen who is better informed regarding health matters, a generally higher standard of living, the better education of youth and the problem of the aged who are surviving in greater numbers than ever before all add to the complexity of the situation. Rising health costs and the sheer number of patients/clients seeking health care also strain our reserves.

Where, then, does the nurse administrator fit into this conglomeration of health care? If it is conceded that the basic function of administration is to serve, then the role of the nurse administrator becomes clearer. The nurse serves her patients, this is true. Thus to a certain extent any nurse administers – she does not need more than the simple management skills related to her functions of providing quality nursing to those in her care. These basic management skills include using time, equipment and facilities, including medications, to the best of her ability to provide a therapeutic environment in which her nursing skills can be practised.

Soon, however, the nurse assumes responsibility commensurate with her level of knowledge and skill for more and more nursing care. Doubtless the time will come when she assumes charge of a unit or a department. Now her management skills are of greater importance. She must ensure that quality care is given, often by others. She has moved higher up the rung of nursing administration and the next step may well be into the floor supervisor, floor nursing service manager, or clinical teaching role. Her function is further removed from the physical provisions of nursing care, except in supervising and teaching. She becomes a *facilitator* of *care*.

This continues up the hierarchy of administration so that those who occupy posts of principal, or chief matron, or chief nursing officer, or regional organiser of nursing services (or whatever nomenclature is current) are often very remote from the practice situation. In this lies a certain danger, for facilitation of care includes knowledge of the care that should be given and the facilities that are necessary to ensure that it is given. The nurse administrator at this high level must also play a part in the policy-making processes necessary for satisfactory management. It can thus be seen that the nurse administrator has a vital role to play in the health care delivery system, a role that has evolved over the ages and will no doubt continue to do so over the years that lie ahead.

Administration enables individuals in cooperation with other individuals to perform functions that are necessary to achieve a desired objective. The objective of nursing administration is to provide quality nursing care for all who need it. The nurse administrator is there to enable this to happen. The organisation and management strategies employed are not for the benefit of the nurse administrator or the nursing personnel, but those for whom the service exists. Nursing and medicine are not business organisations governed by the profit motive.

Nevertheless, many strategies employed in business administration can be applied to the administration of a hospital or other health care system and thus to nursing administration. It is for this reason that there are courses which teach the nurse administrator the basic principles of organisation and management in general terms and the application of these principles to specific areas. The organisational process that may be involved includes such aspects as the following:

☐ Division of work – who does what, when, where, how and why?
☐ Hierarchial structure, including lines of communication and lines of authority
☐ Measures of control, reports, supervision, checking, ordering, inspection, etc
☐ Delegation of authority
☐ Personnel administration, selection, health, utilisation, education (including updating), staff development, job satisfaction, payment, conditions of work, promotion, etc
☐ Record-keeping, patient, research, personnel, special records, etc
☐ Prevention of medico-legal hazards, safety measures, disaster planning
☐ Consultation with heads of other departments – nursing personnel, etc
☐ Finance, including budgeting, economy, control, etc
☐ Leadership.

Many of these aspects are interdependent or related to one another. What is important is that the nurse administrator sees herself as a *nurse*, a *facilitator of nursing care*, someone who *enables quality nursing care* to occur. She should be intimately concerned with:

☐ revising plans for the provision of nursing care
☐ evaluating nursing care
☐ keeping her finger on the pulse of the service for which she is responsible
☐ constant contact and consultation with her personnel

- ☐ coordinating patient care activities and the clinical practice of nursing
- ☐ revising educational programmes to meet modern needs and knowledge
- ☐ providing in-service education programmes to meet defined specific needs in the service for which she is responsible
- ☐ her own reading, up-dating and education.

Nursing administration is not a separate entity, but an integral part of a larger entity which makes up the health care delivery system whether it occurs in a provincial or state hospital, the clinic service, in promotive and preventive health care systems, or in the school nursing or occupational nursing field.

According to records, management has existed since as early as 1300 BCE. Many writers have produced views on the subject which differ, but have common objectives – getting something done. The management of nursing via nursing administration aims to facilitate nursing practice.

The nurse administrator as a manager of nursing has an important role in the health care system. As long as she remembers that this role has nursing as its core concept, she will not go wrong.

NURSING EDUCATION

Nursing itself is as old as man's history, but nursing education as we know it today is of comparatively recent origin.

Specialised training for the profession of nursing probably began towards the end of the eighteenth century, although as early as 1630 St Vincent de Paul expressed a wish that sisters be taught about nursing. It has been recorded that in 1781 Dr Franz May of Mannheim, Germany, persuaded a number of the authorities responsible for the running of hospitals to provide a series of lectures to a number of groups of nursing attendants. This was, in effect, the beginning of the training of secular nurses in hospitals (Searle, 1965: 135). There was some opposition to this from medical colleagues, who feared that the nurses so trained would take work away from medical practitioners. This statement still has a familiar ring today.

In 1793 an Italian, Professor Sannazaro, published an article in which he pointed out to doctors and hospital authorities that the role of the nurse was of great importance in the care of the sick and pleaded for more understanding of this fact (Searle, 1965: 135), and in 1798 a Dr Valentine Seaman delivered a course of lectures to nurses at New York Hospital.

Dr May, convinced that poor nursing engendered by ignorance was the major cause of the high mortality rate in hospitals, was able to persuade others of the validity of his views and thus of the need for formal training of the nursing attendants in hospitals. So successful was he that in 1799 Heidelberg University asked him to establish a university course for the education of nurses. This was a major milestone in nursing education, for at that time no other country in the world had any formal training for nurses, even of an elementary nature. Any training given was an on-the-job haphazard occurrence. Thus it was in Germany that the first course of formal theoretical and practical instruction was organised. Candidates who completed this course satisfactorily were issued with a certificate. Several other schools of nursing based on this were started in Germany, the deaconess training by the Fliedners of Kaiserwerth being an example. Pastor Fliedner at Kaiserwerth started the deaconess training centre, at which formal courses were organised for nurses, teachers and social workers, in 1833. In 1819 Bishop Grégoire appealed for a system of teaching nurses in France and a doctor writing in *Blackwoods* magazine in 1825 advocated teaching nurses and examining their proficiency. The university course offered at Heidelberg was a formal, systematic course which was followed by a further period of planned in-service education.

Florence Nightingale, who is regarded by many as the pioneer of nursing education, visited Kaiserwerth in 1850 for two weeks. In 1951 she spent three months there. After that she also spent some time with the sisters of the L'Hôtel Dieu in Paris. After the Crimean War a fund was raised to honour Miss Nightingale in some permanent way, and a sum of money of £40 000 was raised for the 'Nightingale Fund' which she administered. With this money the Nightingale School was opened in 1860 at St Thomas' Hospital in London. The aim was to train hospital nurses, to train nurses to train others and to train district nurses to care for the sick poor. Thus began a proud tradition of nursing education in England, which was later to spread to many parts of the world.

When nursing education is considered it must not be forgotten that it is a specialised part of the field of general education and is closely allied to medical education. The field of general education has undergone many changes – in fact until comparatively recently any formal education was limited to the wealthy. It was not until at least the latter part of the nineteenth century that the luxury of education was available to anyone outside the moneyed social classes or, in a few instances, to those with special intellectual gifts who were fortunate enough to have these recognised.

Teaching was confined to lecture, demonstration and private study. The supply and availability of books was limited, and there were very few textbooks as we know them today. Technical skills were passed on from master to apprentice in specific trades or occupations. It was only in the early 1900s that a proper study of learning and methods of learning was undertaken. This study resulted in drastic changes in the ideas about what education entailed and the methods that could be used in education.

General education of the public at large became available only in the latter part of the nineteenth century, and even today there are large numbers of people in the world who have received no formal education at all. Coupled with this are tremendous increases in the total body of knowledge, which is growing by the day. The additions have been made by those who have had the education to enable them to search after what is as yet undiscovered in our universe and beyond. All education is groping its way through this massive accumulation of new knowledge and is searching for new and better methods of imparting knowledge and facilitating learning. Minds have to be trained to think and to probe into the future, as has been man's wont since he first inhabitated the earth. Nursing education is no different – it dare not stand still; it must also be shaped to meet the demands of the future. It must prepare not only its practitioners, but also its own scientists, researchers and educators for today and tomorrow.

When Florence Nightingale established her school of nurse training she was not the first to do so. Institutions of religion had already started training nurses – even the training of deaconesses had a religious connotation. She was not even the first to found a school for lay nurses, for this actually ocurred in Lausanne, Switzerland in 1859. Nevertheless, her influence on nurse training was so great that she is generally regarded as the pioneer of modern secular nursing. Florence Nightingale had to tailor her training system to the existing system of 'voluntary' hospitals in England, where the Matron was already an established hospital official and as such could also be in charge of training. Because of its financial independence the Nightingale school had a unique position not easy to emulate in other schools.

The Nightingale pattern did not always fit the established patterns of hospitals in other countries, nor did it always conform to their customs. The concept of the matron as head of the training school did not always fit into the nursing systems already in existence as it did into those in England. Nevertheless, the pattern established by Florence Nightingale could be adapted to meet different needs.

The Nightingale system

This system envisaged by Florence Nightingale adhered to the following pattern:
- ☐ The matron of the hospital was to have supreme responsibility for:
    - the nursing care of patients
    - nursing personnel
    - nursing training
    - the hospital kitchen, linen room and laundry
    - the domestic staff.

    She was answerable only to the Hospital Board, and not to the medical superintendent.
- ☐ The student nurses had to live in a nurses' home, supervised by a 'home sister'.
- ☐ The theoretical education of the nurse had to include basic sciences.
- ☐ The ward sister, under the Matron's direction, had a two-fold responsibility, namely patient care and teaching the student nurses. The sister in charge of a ward was actually paid an extra allowance in recognition of her essential teaching function.

There were two groups of students in the Nightingale school, namely:
- ☐ the *ordinary* probationers who had a year's training followed by three years' supervised practice and were paid a stipend

- the *educated* probationers who followed a formal curriculum which included:
  - 12 hours of anatomy and surgical nursing
  - 12 hours of physiology and medical nursing
  - 12 hours of chemistry, foods and sanitation
  - talks on ethical and professional subjects (lectures, quizzes, notes, case studies, library work and diaries were required of students).

These students had one year of formal training and two years of supervised practice, and paid fees for their training. This latter group of Nightingale nurses was 'trained to train' as its main function. It is because of this that many St Thomas' nurses were sent out by Miss Nightingale to give advice and help in the founding of training schools. This became the pattern throughout the British Isles and in many of the British colonies, including South Africa.

Miss Nightingale's principles of nursing education included the following:
- A school of nursing should be attached to a medical school and a teaching hospital.
- The nurses' home should be a place where a disciplined way of life prevailed and character could be formed. It must be remembered that at the time the reputation of lay nurses was not good and the Nightingale probationers had to be protected from any possibility of gaining such a reputation. This strict discipline was necessary at the time.
- The matron should bear the responsibility for the nurses' entire education programme, including theoretical and practical teaching and experience, and should control the nurses' home, including its rules and regulations.

This pattern is easily discernible in our early education of nurses. Many South Africans still use the term matron, although it is falling into disuse even in Britain. In South Africa the official term is now 'nursing service manager'.

The American system

This is an adaptation of the Nightingale system and is found in Canada, the United States of America and other countries. Its main features include the following:
- Training schools are attached to hospitals. The superintendent of nurses is responsible for patient care, the term matron not being used except for a housekeeper type of grade.
- A dietician controls the catering department and its personnel (this is another area where changes are occurring throughout the world).
- A housekeeper or 'matron' controls the domestic department.
- The superintendent of nurses is responsible to the Board or the superintendent of the hospital, who could be a doctor, a nurse or a layman.
- Students live in a nurses' home or outside.
- The theoretical instruction is very broadly based.

- 'Head nurse' is the term used to denote the person in charge of a ward. A 'supervisor' is in charge of a department consisting of several wards. She is responsible for teaching and disciplining students and for the management of the wards in her department.

Other systems include the following:

The Motherhouse system

This is a modern adaptation of that developed by the old religious orders. It is found in the parts of the world where a school is maintained by a religious sisterhood, Catholic or Protestant, as well as in the Red Cross schools of Switzerland and Germany. The theoretical instruction may be quite elementary, the ward sister has an important teaching function, and sisters are supported for life, living in a nurses' home.

The Continental system

Found all over the European continent and in Latin America, the Continental system exists side by side with the Motherhouse system and has adopted certain features from both the Nightingale system and the American system. There is, however, no equivalent of the 'matron' or the superintendent of nurses. Each 'service' block (eg medical nursing) has its own head nurse who is directly responsible to a doctor in charge of the 'block' and also to the director of the hospital, who may be a layman or a doctor.

The training school may form an integral part of the hospital or it may be an independent educational institution. Theoretical instruction is given and students are given practical instruction by various means. They are supernumerary in the wards. The role of the ward sister in teaching also varies. In the early days training was hampered by the illiteracy of the masses. This improved with the increased availability of general education.

In most countries today there are at least three systems of basic education of the nurse:

- The preparation for professional practice with registration of qualifications. This may be offered at baccalaureate, associate degree or diploma (or in some countries at certificate) level.
- Preparation of a subprofessional level of nurse who is usually prepared for enrolment or licensure at hospital training schools.
- Preparation of a group of qualified assistants to the two first categories. These are nurses' assistants or assistant nurses who assist registered and/or enrolled nurses.

The programmes offered vary throughout the world and changes and adaptations are constantly being made. Courses vary with regard to duration and admission requirements and in many countries students pay for their training. Basic university education for nurses is accepted in the United States of America, Belgium, Great Britain, New Zealand, Canada, Israel and South

Africa. Other countries are working towards this. In countries where nursing degrees are not available, nurse leaders often study the arts, social sciences, philosophy or economics at degree level.

The development of nursing education in South Africa

Sister Henrietta Stockdale introduced nurse training into South Africa when she instituted a training programme at the Carnarvon Hospital in Kimberley in 1877. Lectures for the first group commenced in February 1877. A ward for Black patients at the Digger's Central Hospital as well as the wards of the Carnarvon Hospital were used for practical training purposes. Later these two hospitals were united to form the Kimberley Hospital.

The first training course was one year in duration, the knowledge obtained being tested by examination. The students had to serve another year as staff nurses before they gained recognition as trained nurses. Eminent medical men assisted greatly in the training programme. Sister Henrietta was a great advocate of nursing education being part of the general education system of the country, but unfortunately for the progress of nursing education in this country she had little success in this area and the struggle continues to this day. Just recently, with the colleges of nursing in cooperation with universities being responsible for basic registered nurse training, this ideal is being realised.

The part of the training programme which is interesting in the light of later developments is that the lectures were concentrated in the winter months. A 'block' system in embryo? Subjects included anatomy, physiology, practical nursing, surgery and sick cookery. Ethical instruction was also given. A second course of lectures was included in the second year while nurses were serving as staff nurses and a second examination was conducted towards the end of the second year. Thus theoretical and clinical instruction was combined with practical experience. Kimberley-trained nurses, much like the Nightingale nurses in Britain, spread their influence far and wide and, among others, started training nurses at Barberton in 1877, at the Volkshospitaal Pretoria in 1890, and at the Frontier Hospital, Queenstown, in 1890. Sister Henrietta also helped Sister Mary Agatha to start training at the Somerset Hospital in 1886, when three ladies of 'education and refinement' were admitted as probationers.

By the end of the nineteenth century there were eighteen hospitals in South Africa where the training of nurses was undertaken and a Kimberley-trained nurse was associated with each of these training schools. This was no mean achievement! The examination of nurses became the responsibility of the Colonial Medical Council in 1892. Prior to this examinations were conducted by the hospitals themselves. The first Afrikaans woman to train as a nurse was Alice Eveline de Beer (1886). The educational requirements laid down by Sister Henrietta for admission to training were that prospective students should be 'cultured young women' who understood the three Rs thoroughly, had read widely, knew Latin, and played some musical instrument. So highly was the training at Kimberley valued that educated women had their names entered on a waiting list and some had to wait as long as five years for admission to training. At the same time it must be remembered that the number admitted to training at any one time was small. Nurses in training at Kimberley Hospital were supernumerary and paid a fee for tuition.

From small beginnings come great developments. The examination and certification of nurses was taken over by the various medical councils as they became established, until the passage of the *Medical, Dental and Pharmacy Act,* 1928 (Act 13 of 1928), when the South African Medical Council came into being. This provided for recognition of the certificates issued and the registration of nurses granted by the various medical councils. The South African Medical Council became the registering body for midwives and nurses, with disciplinary powers and powers to approve training schools, to conduct examinations and to grant certificates. It also provided for recognition of additional qualifications.

By the time the South African Medical Council assumed responsibility for nurse training the training period was three years in Class I training schools and four years in Class II training schools. Unfortunately for the education of the nurse, Sister Henrietta's plan for nursing education as part of general education was not implemented and an apprenticeship system of training which greatly exploited the students and from which we have not yet entirely escaped was introduced. Lectures were given only as examination time drew near and in the students off-duty time. Nurses were taught *how* to do something, but seldom *why*. Such practice was against the Nightingale and the Stockdale principles of how nursing education should take place.

In 1937 the South African Medical Council increased the training period to three-and-a-half years and four-and-a-half years for Class I and Class II training schools respectively. In 1921 a preliminary training school system was introduced at the Johannesburg Hospital, to which the first qualified sister tutor in South Africa, Miss MEG Milne, was appointed in October of that year. In June 1932 Miss EM Pike established a full block system at Groote Schuur Hospital. After a period of struggle for professional control of nurses by nurses, the Nursing Act was passed in 1944. This established the South African Nursing Council (SANC) which took over responsibility from the South African Medical Council for the examination and registration of nurses and for the approval of training schools. It had disciplinary powers and could lay down training programmes, syllabusses and the educational requirements for entry. It also recognised post-basic qualifications.

When the South African Nursing Council took over these responsibilities in 1944 the apprenticeship system of training was still in force except at Groote Schuur Hospital, where the 'block' system was used. Gradually changes were brought about. The hours of practice were reduced, lectures were given in 'duty' time, and students were less exploited. In 1945 there were only 29 trained sister tutors in the Union of South Africa, of whom six were able to teach in Afrikaans. In 1986, 41 years later, there was a total of 2 068 on the register, of whom 1 489 were White, 144 Coloured, 37 Indian and 698 Black.

It is realised that not all those on the register are actively engaged in teaching. Nevertheless an improvement is obvious, although the numbers are still too small and there is a great maldistribution among the races to meet their own needs. It must be remembered that basic nursing education among the Coloured, Indian and Black groups on a large scale is of recent origin, and a great deal of teaching in Non-White training schools is still done by White tutors.

More and more teachers are being prepared for nursing education in all race groups and in 1975 the increase of 40 Black registered tutors out of a total of 52 new registrations was encouraging. In 1986 the number of Black registered tutors increased by 64 out of a total increase of 179 (from 1985-1986). In 1945 the educational standard required to be admitted to training for registration was only Standard VII. Today it is Standard X (12 years of schooling). The practical training hours required by the South African Medical Council in Class I training schools was 8 664 and the minimum number of hours of lectures prescribed was 100 plus 100 demonstrations. It must be pointed out that the minimum was seldom exceeded. Today a minimum of clinical practica and a minimum of lecture periods (theoretical instruction) is laid down for the education of a registered nurse.

Some of the historical information is broadly based on sections of Searle 1965: ch 19.

The period of training to be undergone for basic registration is now four years. The training of singly qualified midwives has been stopped. Midwifery training for the registered nurse increased from six months to nine months, and then to one year, except where the comprehensive approach is used.

Recent developments

A significant development of recent years was the advent in 1969 of the integrated course combining general nursing and midwifery.

The comprehensive course

Regulations for the comprehensive course were promulgated on 30 September 1983. This course covers at least four academic years and includes General Nursing Science, Psychiatric Nursing Science, Midwifery and Community Nursing Science. The course will eventually phase out other courses, since the regulations state that 'no person may, after 1 January 1986, be registered as a student at a nursing school for the first time, unless he registers for the course referred to in these regulations' (Government Notice no. R2118).

This is an exciting development in nursing education in South Africa. Nursing schools will be linked with universities and nursing education is thus clearly regarded as part of the tertiary education system of the country. The status of nursing colleges will be in no doubt and student status will be more readily understood. This does not mean that student nurses will not participate in patient care, but that their learning needs will be taken into consideration at all times. The change should ultimately produce a better registered nurse capable of contributing to the improvement of nursing, and thus health care, at all levels.

* * *

The South African Nursing Council constantly reviews training programmes and new regulations are made after careful consideration and consultation with experts in the different fields. Many factors have to be taken into account when regulations are framed. These include:
- [ ] the needs of the public for well-trained persons in all categories to supply nursing care of a high standard
- [ ] the educational needs of students and pupils
- [ ] admission requirements which will ensure that the educational programme objectives will be met and which are at the same time realistic
- [ ] the necessity to tailor training regulations flexibly enough so that they can be adapted to meet constantly changing needs created by new techniques employed in nursing and medical practice.

The South African Nursing Council issues directives which are constantly under review to training schools. These set out the purpose of the courses, the course content and the minimum qualification of lecturers as well as the minimum number of teaching periods required. Because they are not embodied in regulations, the amendment of which takes considerable time, they are easily altered. Regulations are framed in very broad terms; directives include more details.

The South African Nursing Council registers general nurses, midwives, psychiatric nurses and now also community nurses after completion of a prescribed period of training and the passing of examinations. Similarly, it enrols nurses after shorter, less intensive training and also enrols nursing assistants who have a still shorter period of training which is mostly practical in nature. It also registers additional qualifications after the student has followed either a course prescribed by the South African Nursing Council and passed its examination, or followed a course of study and passed an examination conducted by another institution which has been approved by the Council for that purpose. Education in the following specialities is now possible:
- [ ] Nursing Education
- [ ] Nursing Administration
- [ ] Community Nursing Science
- [ ] Paediatric Nursing Science
- [ ] Orthopaedic Nursing Science
- [ ] Operating Theatre Nursing Science
- [ ] Ophthalmic Nursing Science
- [ ] Spinal Injury Nursing Science
- [ ] Oncology Nursing Science

- [ ] Geriatric Nursing Science
- [ ] Occupational Health Nursing
- [ ] Clinical Nursing Science, Health Assessment, Treatment and Care
- [ ] Renal Nursing.

Community Nursing Science is now becoming a basic qualification, although the many thousands of registered nurses who do not yet have this qualification can still complete the post-registration course. Advanced courses in many areas of nursing specialisation are now available.

The first nursing college was established at the Johannesburg General Hospital in 1945. Today there are many throughout the country. University education for nurses began with the establishment of courses leading to the Diploma in Nursing (Tutor) at the universities of the Witwatersrand and Cape Town, which admitted the first students in 1937. The first six students to complete the course obtained their diplomas at the University of the Witwatersrand on 11 March 1939. In 1949 the University of Pretoria instituted a one-year diploma course for tutors. This was the first course offered through the medium of Afrikaans.

Other universities have followed suit. In 1956 the University of Natal instituted the first course specifically for Non-White sister tutors. The University of the North offers a similar course. Of course some Non-White students obtained diplomas in Nursing Education at other universities and the Transvaal ran a tutor's course based at Baragwanath Hospital for a short time. The Diploma in Hospital Administration was pioneered by Professor C Searle, then directress of Nursing Services of the Transvaal Administration at the Pretoria College of Nursing. This course, too, has now moved into universities and in some cases is offered in combination with Community Nursing.

A basic degree course for nurses was introduced at the University of Pretoria in 1956. The first was a four-and-a-half-year programme leading to a BA Nursing. This course has undergone changes. It is now a four-and-a-half-year course for the degree Baccalaureus Curationis (BCur) and follows the integrated approach so that students obtain registration as general nurses, midwives and psychiatric nurses. Students who have followed this course have proceeded to further study. A master's degree (MCur) is available in nursing education, nursing administration, clinical nursing and other fields and there have already been several graduates from this programme. A doctorate, the DCur, is also available and to date there have been several graduates.

Other universities have followed the University of Pretoria and now offer nursing degrees ranging from BCur, BSc (Nursing), BASc (Nursing), BSoc Sc, and others.

Basic (generic) nursing degrees are also offered at Medunsa and, in the independent states, at the University of Fort Hare. Other universities in these states offer post-registration diplomas and degrees for registered nurses. Most of the universities offer post-graduate courses and have graduates from these programmes.

The degree BCur (I et A) was introduced at the University of Pretoria in 1970. The (I et A) stands for *Institutionis et Administrationis*, that is Education and Administration and the course was designed to meet the needs of registered nurses who did not qualify by means of a basic degree. It enabled them, in a minimum period of three years, to obtain registration as nurse educators and nurse administrators, and in some cases also as community nurses, at the same time as obtaining a degree. Other universities offer similar courses. It is one of the most valuable courses available at present, because it enables nurses who can obtain their basic qualification only by diploma courses to study in depth while obtaining post-basic qualifications. This course is also available at the University of the North, a university for Black students.

The inception by the University of South Africa of degree and diploma courses in nursing at post-registration level has opened up the field to nurses of all races with the necessary nursing and educational qualifications. The degree known as the BA(Cur) was instituted in 1976. Honours, masters and doctoral programmes are also available. This means that students who cannot attend a residential university can also study for a degree and obtain registration in nursing education, or in nursing administration or community nursing. Many students are availing themselves of this opportunity, and there have been a number of graduates from the programmes and from postgraduate programmes up to doctoral level. Some universities have separated the Masters courses into Honours courses and a research Masters.

The training of the subprofessional groups (the enrolled nurse, whose course is of two years' duration, and the enrolled nursing assistant, who follows a short practical course of 100 days and works under the supervision, direct or indirect, of the registered nurse) ensures that health care is available at all levels and adds to the nursing force in our country. The training and examination of these groups is also controlled by the South African Nursing Council.

Nursing in South Africa is a closed profession. No person may practise any form of nursing for gain unless she is registered or enrolled with the South African Nursing Council. This measure is aimed at protecting the public. Ethical control is exercised over all registered and enrolled persons and nursing education extends to all who practise nursing for gain. The type of course varies for the different categories of worker, but it is controlled.

Nursing education in South Africa is dynamic. It changes constantly to keep pace with the needs of medicine and nursing and patients and clients, and is ready to adapt and alter its programmes continually. It takes cognisance of changes in general education and adapts its techniques to its own needs. The trend towards a better-educated, thinking nurse who acts with considered judgement to fulfil her role is just as much part of the nursing education pattern in the Republic as it is in other parts of the world. Remember that, as Florence Nightingale is reported to have said, the nurse who stands still goes backward.

The need for continuing education is recognised and met by post-registration courses as well as in-service programmes. The latter will have to be expanded and organised to meet felt as well as observed needs, but they are there and can be extended.

11 The concept 'health' in the nursing context

The World Health Organisation's definition of health is too well known to require reiteration. It is an extremely positive concept. Nevertheless the nurse, like any other health professional, realises that the meaning of health is relative and has a different import for different people. Some people regard very slight deviations from a *perceived* standard of health as catastrophic, while others accept quite marked deviations as *good health*.

Nursing is involved in restoring health to people and assisting them to maintain and promote health. The very use of the word 'promote' in a health context implies that there are variations in the state of health and that a so-called 'well' person can actually become 'more well'. The emphasis is on 'wholeness' of the mind and body.

Health is thus a highly individual concept; it is dynamic, in a constant state of change. A deviation from a state of health, ill-health, even 'illness' means that the individual no longer feels 'well'. His feelings may vary from vague discomfort to acute distress. The experience of illness, the feeling of 'not being well', is highly individual and may not be related to an actual pathological state in the person 'feeling unwell'. Some states of deviation from health will cause an individual to be unable to function − severe haemorrhaging will cause collapse and death if untreated. On the other hand, it is difficult to judge the intensity of a headache − at various stages in an individual's life the pain of such a condition may cause him to be quite incapacitated, while at others he may continue to function fairly satisfactorily.

An individual formulates his own perception of acceptable forms of behaviour relating to illness in accordance with familial and other cultural norms. Religious beliefs also determine acceptance of suffering and responses to deviations from health. The nurse, herself culturally conditioned with regard to health matters, formulates her own perception of appropriate behaviour in those suffering from ill-health.

In the course of her nursing ministrations a nurse will encounter many people from different backgrounds in which different norms pertain and who exhibit quite different reactions to similar health problems. Her concern must always be with the *person*, with what he is and what he does. Observation of behaviours, observation that is as free as is humanly possible of preconceived expectations, will help her to meet health needs. Acceptance of the person for whom she is caring as a person in need of the type of care that she is trained to give, is vital. Her interpretations of the signs and symptoms that she observes must not be clouded by the behaviour 'expected' of someone according to her personal frame of reference. Overt as well as covert behaviour must be observed and interpreted. Vital signs can be measured, behaviour in the face of them cannot.

The nurse is also a human being, with human frailties and fallibility. She has her own problems and anxieties. Her personal reactions to health service problems may be difficult to conceal and may transfer from one episode to another. It is only when the nurse realises that this is a feature of any nursing situation and that she has to face her own problems realistically in order to meet the needs of others that she really matures professionally.

Nurses have their own ideas about what a 'good nurse' should say and do. These ideas may be built on false premises and on generalisations about the concept health and its meaning to others. Patients also have preconceived ideas concerning appropriate behaviour on the part of nurses. It would be as well for nurses to determine what these are and whether they are actually retarding recovery by completely negating a patient's ideas of 'what a good nurse' does. A realistic examination of her own ideas about health and health service in relation to patient needs and conceptions may lead to a reappraisal of appropriate behaviour, to the benefit of all concerned.

SICKNESS AND SOCIETY

The sick person, as a member of society, must be viewed in terms of his relationship to that society. First he is a member of a family, functioning in different social roles as a well member of that family, of his community and thus of society.

A deviation from a state of health disrupts this pattern. It is like a performance of a stage play. A minor deviation like a headache may cause an actor to play badly and may upset and even irritate fellow actors if the whole performance is affected. They may be sorry for their fellow actor, but no major disruption occurs. Let the same actor fall and break an ankle and the whole pattern changes. He will receive a great deal of sympathy, but he will have to be replaced. An understudy will have to play his part, extra rehearsals will have to be called, and reorganisation will be necessary. If it happens an hour before the start of a performance even more choas may occur. 'The show must go on!' But how? A major deviation has occurred.

Illness can disrupt a family (especially if the victim is the breadwinner), the work situation or have quite far-reaching consequences for society as a whole. The patient has an illness and this is a crisis in his life as an individual. If he is the only mathematics teacher available in a school and his disease is serious, the repercussions may be widespread. It may disrupt the teaching programme so much that his scholars are seriously handicapped. If some should fail their end of year examinations because of a lack of teaching it might adversely affect their future careers. Thus a sick person does not affect only himself.

Society does not view sickness as a desirable state of affairs. At the same time changes in society occur which alter the pattern of disease and new health needs arise. New habits, new customs and changes in population, its grouping and location cause new health problems, which are continuous. Urbanisation brought the diseases of community living to the fore and created needs for proper sanitation, the safe disposal of refuse and an uncontaminated water and food supply for the inhabitants of towns. Housing of a standard that did not encourage disease-spreading or disease-producing conditions had to be provided. Thus society and its changes can cause ill-health.

Similarly society can, if its social conscience is aroused, do much to prevent disease and alleviate suffering. Attitudes to sickness and suffering are largely culturally determined. Although the knowledge relating to health and health care, including the prevention of sickness, may exist, unless society adopts sound health practices based on the existing knowledge of sickness, 'ill-health' will prevail. Theoretically, today medical knowledge is available to the whole world. Science is supposed to know no barriers and yet, despite the work of the World Health Organisation, individual governments and dedicated health professionals, two thirds of the inhabitants of the earth still die from disease conditions that are preventable.

Despite the knowledge available, sickness – that is preventable sickness – will continue to flourish where economic pressures and the lack of trained health service personnel render the provision of health care inadequate to meet the needs of the population. Man-made conditions such as wars and terrorism and natural disasters such as floods and earthquakes also wreak havoc on the equilibrium necessary in man's environment if he is to enjoy good health. The social changes that have occurred as a result of decreases in infant mortality and increased longevity have also brought about changes in the type of health care needed. From perambulator manufacture to wheelchair manufacture in the course of less than a century may well be a reality in the more developed countries!

The provision of modern health care facilities is extremely expensive. It is only the society that has enough wealth among its members that can afford such luxuries as modern, well-equipped hospitals staffed with highly trained health professionals of all categories. Medical research is also extremely expensive. Fortunately, the results of expensive research can be applied universally.

There are many aspects of sickness and society that are beyond the scope of this particular work. Some societies have provided for health needs by means such as national insurance, medical aid schemes, the National Health Service of Britain and welfare services of various types. Because of the complicated nature of the treatment of the diseases that are prevalent in developed countries and the expense involved, it is sound economic sense to prevent as much ill-health as possible, but how much of the national budget of a country should be devoted to health services, preventive, promotive or curative? This is something that only society itself can decide upon. Nurses, as members of society, can only act in accordance with their own lights.

Perhaps they can stir social conscience to the realisation that money spent on prevention is money saved. They can do this only if they themselves realise the truth of this statement and talk and act with authority based on firm conviction.

MEDICAL CRISES AND THE NURSE

Crisis – a moment of danger or suspense. When the danger is of a medical nature, the health of a patient hangs in the balance. Medical crises may be completely unexpected or there may be warning signs. There are some disease conditions that are more liable to episodes of crisis than others. Some will be fatal.

Where does the nurse fit into this pattern? Obviously her trained observation and judgement must be brought into play to prevent crises from developing or to deal with those that have already occurred. In order to prevent a crisis from developing or to minimise its potentially fatal effect it is necessary to know what dangers are inherent in a disease, the signs and symptoms that precede the actual crisis situation and the preventive measures that must be taken by the nurse, the patient and sometimes the members of a patient's family. A case in point is a patient suffering from diabetes mellitus. Two situations potentially extremely dangerous to life may develop, namely a hyperglycaemic coma or a hypoglycaemic coma. The education of the nurse will include all aspects of the pre-recognition, prevention and appropriate treatment to prevent the development of a coma. Furthermore, she will learn how to teach the patient and, where necessary, his family what to do and what not to do to avoid such crises.

Many other medical conditions in which there are such dangers come to mind. Cardiac conditions, haemophilia, severe allergies and epilepsy are some of them. If in these impending or actual crises signs are not read properly, or are read too slowly, the patient may be in danger of losing his life, being permanently disabled or coming dangerously near to death. Mistakes can occur – all health care personnel are human – but careful attention to observation, to teaching and preparation, to assessment of the situation and to action based on knowledge and educated judgement can do much to minimise these.

Similarly, knowledge of the basic principles of care can be of immense value in dealing with unexpected crisis situations such as an unexpected gastric haemorrhage, a perforated duodenal ulcer in a patient previously free of symptoms, a sudden myocardial infarct, a cardiac arrest or a person collapsing at work or play. In these crises the nurse who knows the simple rules regarding positioning, maintaining an open airway and resuscitation techniques can do much to help the patient until more sophisticated means can be employed. The nurse must not only *know* how to act in a medical crisis, she must also actually *carry out* the appropriate action and be able to *guide others* to assist and give emotional support to the patient and his family.

A nurse does not stand helpless in the face of medical crises. She uses her trained ability to deal as competently as she can with the situation until further aid is available.

CHRONIC ILLNESS AND THE NURSE

The nurse has a tremendous role to play in the management of chronic illness. Her acceptance of the sick person as a human being with dignity despite his ailment can do much to assist the patient in coming to terms with his affliction and finding some meaning in the limited faculties that are left to him.

The problems faced by a person adjusting to a chronic illness (and, indeed, of his family, in the midst of whom he must live) must be perceived. The patient may come into hospital for acute episodes, but he has a family to whom he returns, a home in which he lives. Those suffering from a chronic illness have many problems that are not real to those who have not experienced them. Mobility, or rather the lack thereof, is a case in point. Assistance with financial problems, the reorganisation of his physical environment to help the patient to cope with the essentials of daily life and the necessary supportive services, social contacts outside the home and daily treatment are all aspects of the management of chronic illness. The nurse in the community sees more of this than the hospital-based nurse, but a little thought on the part of the latter before her patients' discharge so that suitable channels of help can be contacted can do much to alleviate the lot of the chronically ill.

THE RIGHTS AND RESPONSIBILITIES OF THE NURSE

To conclude this exposition on the ethos of nursing it would be as well to pause briefly and consider the nurse of today against the background of her place in society and her rights and responsibilities.

A look at the Declaration of Human Rights will point out very clearly that rights can be spelt out for all without pointing out any reciprocal responsibilities relating to the recipients of those rights. This book has moved far in the other direction. The duties of a nurse have been discussed in some detail, accountability in the nursing profession has received attention and discipline and nursing and the need for self-discipline have come under scrutiny. The aim of all nursing has been shown to be service to other human beings and the nurse's responsibilities in various situations have been spelt out.

In all this the nurse has been shown to have many responsibilities, but little mention has been made of her rights. A nurse is also a human being entitled to live a full life, to proper education for her role, to a just wage for her work and to working conditions and conditions of service which enable her to give the quality care for which she is prepared and to derive job satisfaction from her work. The nurse is entitled to consideration of her needs and feelings and a place in the sun of daily living.

Nursing is a caring profession, but the nurse, in turn, should also receive a measure of caring for her rights from the public and her employers so that she can meet her many responsibilities with confidence and enthusiasm. Study of the ethos of nursing might well give more meaning to its practice.

Let nursing go forward into the future secure in the knowledge that a good foundation has been laid in the past and in the present. It is up to nurses to realise the full potential inherent in their profession. The future is theirs.

Appendices

A THE HIPPOCRATIC OATH

- ☐ I swear by Apollo the healer, by Aesculapius, by Health and all the powers of healing, and call to witness all the gods and goddesses that I may keep this oath and promise to the best of my ability and judgement.
- ☐ I will pay the same respect to my master in the science as to my parents and share my life with him and pay all my debts to him. I will regard his sons as my brothers and teach them the science, if they desire to learn it without fee or contract. I will hand on precepts, lectures and all other learnings to my sons, to those of my master and to those pupils duly appointed and sworn, and to none other.
- ☐ I will use my powers to help the sick to the best of my ability and judgement; I will abstain from harming or wronging any man by it.
- ☐ I will not give a fatal draught to anyone if I am asked, nor will I suggest any such thing. Neither will I give a woman means to procure an abortion.
- ☐ I will be chaste and religious in my life and in my practice.
- ☐ I will not cut, even for the stone, but I will leave such procedures to the practitioners of that craft.
- ☐ Whenever I go into a house, I will go to help the sick and never with intention of doing harm or injury. I will not abuse my position to indulge in sexual contacts with the bodies of women or of men, whether they be freemen or slaves.
- ☐ Whatever I see or hear, whether professionally or privately, which ought not to be divulged, I will keep secret and tell no one.
- ☐ If, therefore, I observe this oath and do not violate it, may I prosper both in my life and in my profession earning good repute among all men for all time. If I transgress and forswear this oath, may my lot be otherwise.

B PRACTICAL IMPLICATIONS OF THE HEALTH ACT FOR NURSING

The establishment of a National Health Policy Council

'The aim of this Council is to ensure that the various authorities which provide health services in the Republic shall carry out all such activities as they are authorised to do under the Health Act and any other applicable law, "to promote the health of the inhabitants of the Republic so that every person shall be enabled to attain and maintain a state of complete physical, mental and social well-being, and which shall exercise such other powers and perform such other duties as may be conferred or imposed upon it by this Act"' (Searle, *Aspects of community health*, p. 29).

The constitution of this Council provides for a Minister of Health and members of the Executive Committee of each province, who are charged with Hospital Services. Thus is is possible to put the health problems specific to any province or area in that province directly to the government of the day. The secretary of this Council is the Secretary of Health. 'The function of the Council essentially is to consider recommendations made by the Health Matters Advisory Committee to the Minister in regard to the formulation of a national policy in regard to the rendering of health services by the Department of Health and Welfare, provincial administrations and local authorities, and health services generally' (Strauss, *Legal handbook for nurses and health personnel*, p. 88).

Although nurses are not directly involved in this Council it is essential that they know it exists and understand its function, as will become clear from the next paragraph.

The Health Matters Advisory Committee

This Committee is of vital importance. It is composed of representatives of the Department of Health and Welfare, including the Director-General, the Director of Hospital Services of each provincial administration, Medical Officers of Health of local authorities rendering services in urban as well as rural areas, and the Surgeon-General of the South African Defence Force. The Committee considers health matters and makes recommendations to the National Health Advisory Council.

One of the most important implications of this Health Matters Advisory Committee for all health professionals, and thus for nurses, is that it is assisted in the performance of its duties by various subcommittees which have *expert* knowledge in their respective fields.

The practical implications for nursing practice are that one of the subcommittees which has been appointed is the Subcommittee on Nursing. This Committee consists of representatives of the Department of Health and Welfare, the South African Military Nursing Service, the Department of Prisons, the four provincial Departments of Hospital Services, local authorities and the South African Nursing Association.

With the exception of the Chairman, who must be a member of the Health Matters Advisory Committee, all the members of the Subcommittee on Nursing are nurses and thus represent a wide spectrum of nursing services and of expertise and interests. Already the Subcommittee on Nursing has had an impact on nursing practice by providing meaningful input regarding nursing salaries and conditions of service, but its influence extends far beyond this. The Committee is concerned with the totality of nursing and nursing services.

The appointment of the Subcommittee means that, for the first time, nurses have a major role to play at the policy-making level of government. They consider matters related to nursing in depth and make recommendations to the Health Matters Advisory Committee. This Committee, in turn, makes recommendations to the National Health Policy Council.

It may seem that the new dispensation is rather far removed from the average professional nurse in practice, but the members of the Subcommittee on Nursing have the fullest right to consult any member of the profession, at any level, for advice or information on specific aspects of the rendering of nursing services. This power or right is spelt out in the provisions of the functions of the Health Matters Advisory Committee, which states: 'the committee may at its discretion, in regard to any matter falling within the scope of its functions, consult any person, body or authority and may take evidence from or hear representations by such person, body or authority' (section 3 (2) of the Health Act). The same provisions apply to the members of the subcommittees. Thus the members of the Subcommittee on Nursing can also institute inquiry into specific problem areas. This type of inquiry or investigation could involve many nurses, even though only by completing a simple questionnaire. It is also possible for nurses to bring specific problem areas to the attention of the members of the Subcommittee, who then have a truly broad base of relevant information upon which to debate and base their recommendations regarding policy.

This direct advisory function of the Subcommittee on Nursing to the Health Matters Advisory Committee has an important practical implication for nursing which emanates from the Health Act.

Registered nurses also serve on other subcommittees besides the Subcommittee on Nursing and are thus able to put forward the nursing point of view and make a valuable contribution to not only the health services as such, but also the future planning of such services. The framework for full participation by nurses now exists, and it is being used.

Other important aspects of the Health Act are that it lays down clearly the functions of the following:

The various Departments of Health and Welfare

The functions of the Departments of Health and Welfare include:
- ☐ the coordination of health services rendered by the Departments, with due regard to health services rendered by provincial administrations and local authorities
- ☐ the establishment of a national health laboratory service
- ☐ promotion of a safe and healthy environment
- ☐ the promotion of family planning
- ☐ the provision of services for the procurement of evaluation of evidence of a medical nature with a view to legal proceedings
- ☐ any other functions as may be assigned to it by the Minister.

The practical implications for nurses, especially those employed by the Departments, are thus related to assisting in the coordination of services and the promotion of family planning, as well as undertaking or participating in relevant research programmes.

The provincial administrations

The functions of the provincial administrations include:
- ☐ the provision of hospital facilities and services

- the provision of an ambulance service within its province and, where necessary, the coordination of services with adjacent provincial services
- the provision of facilities for the treatment of patients suffering from acute mental illness
- the provision of out-patient facilities in hospitals or other places where patients are treated for a period of less than 24 hours
- the provision of maternity homes and services
- the provision of personal health services, either on its own or in cooperation with local authorities
- the coordination of services with a view to the establishment of a comprehensive health service in the province, taking into account the services rendered by others providing health services
- any other functions assigned to it by the Minister.

Here the practical implications for nursing practice are perhaps more obvious, as the nurse is heavily involved in rendering nursing care and supplying nursing services at a visible level.

The Act indicates that the function of the provincial administrations shall be to provide certain facilities or services, but does not actually state that they themselves render such services. This means that the facilities of other existing organisations may continue to be used, being duly compensated monetarily therefore by the provincial administration budget.

From a nursing point of view this means that much closer cooperation between services is possible and that the services should no longer consider their functions in separate 'compartments'. It should also make it possible to assess the services being rendered by the various authorities and thus to eliminate unnecessary duplication.

Another factor to be considered is that the provincial authorities can become involved in more primary health care centres where patients are not accommodated overnight and in incorporating immunisation services and family planning clinics into their existing hospital out-patient or detached clinics. This is already being done, but with more careful consultation and planning among the various authorities much more coordination could be achieved, which would benefit patients and clients and ensure the prudent allocation of scarce resources, both human and material.

Local authorities

The functions of the local authorities include:
- the maintenance of its district in a clean and hygienic condition at all times
- the prevention of the occurrence of any nuisance within its district
- when a nuisance has occurred, abating it or causing it to be abated, or remedying it or causing it to be remedied
- preventing the pollution of water intended for the use of the inhabitants of its district
- the prevention of communicable diseases, the promotion of the health of persons, and the rehabilitation in the community of persons cured of any medical conditions and participation in the coordination of such services.

A nuisance is defined and other provisions are laid down, including aspects such as the appointment of medical officers of health, nurses, health inspectors and other health personnel.

Provisions are also made for the making of regulations which add flesh to the skeleton provided by the Act with which to carry out the intentions of the Act without it being necessary to resort to amendments of the Act each time – a quite impractical state of affairs.

Again it can be seen that there is provision for the coordination of health services, which has very obvious implications for nursing practice.

In November 1980 the Minister of Health announced that a National Health Services Facilities Plan had been drawn up. This plan was formulated by the Subcommittee for Health Service Buildings and submitted to the Health Matters Advisory Committee. This Committee, in turn, placed the matter before the National Health Policy Council, which approved the plan. Thus it is clear that the coordinative system instituted by the Health Act does play a role in the formulation of policy which should not be underestimated.

The underlying principle of the National Health Services Facilities Plan is the need for a policy which provides not only for *facilities*, but for the *actual delivery* of health services and *the provision of funds* for the development of a comprehensive service.

Other principles incorporated in the plan are the following:
☐ Centralisation of policy formation and planning of health services, facilities and strategy
☐ Decentralisation of services and facilities in which the promotive, preventive, rehabilitative and curative components all take their rightful place
☐ Shifting of emphasis from a curatively oriented service to a service in which attention is also given to basic needs, the promotion of health and other facets of health care
☐ Community involvement
☐ Coordination of services and collective utilisation of facilities by different authorities
☐ Recognition of the task of the private practitioner and the integration of his services with those of the public sector.

The above has been a brief summary of the provisions of the Health Act and the reader is referred to the Act itself, to Searle and Brink (*Aspects of community health*), or to Strauss (*Legal handbook for nurses and health personnel*) for more information.

For those practising in other countries or in the national states, it is suggested that you study the legislation pertaining to the country or state in which you work, with particular reference to the nursing implications.

C THE NATIONAL HEALTH PLAN*

This plan was formulated in 1986 with the aim of achieving a comprehensive health service for South Africa. It sees the essential perspectives regarding health as:
☐ a centralised policy for achieving national health goals and priorities

* As stated in the brochure 'A New Dispensation; health services in South Africa', obtained from the Department of Health.

- centralised responsibility for the provision of health services
- decentralised implementation based on the National Plan for Health Service Facilities.

It states that the process of rendering comprehensive health services involves:
- the identification of national health objectives and priorities
- acceptance of a national policy to achieve the health objectives in a coordinated manner
- the implementation of the national health policy by means of the *National Health Plan*
- continuous monitoring of the rendering of health services and modification of national health objectives and priorities as called for.

The National Health Plan and associated variables

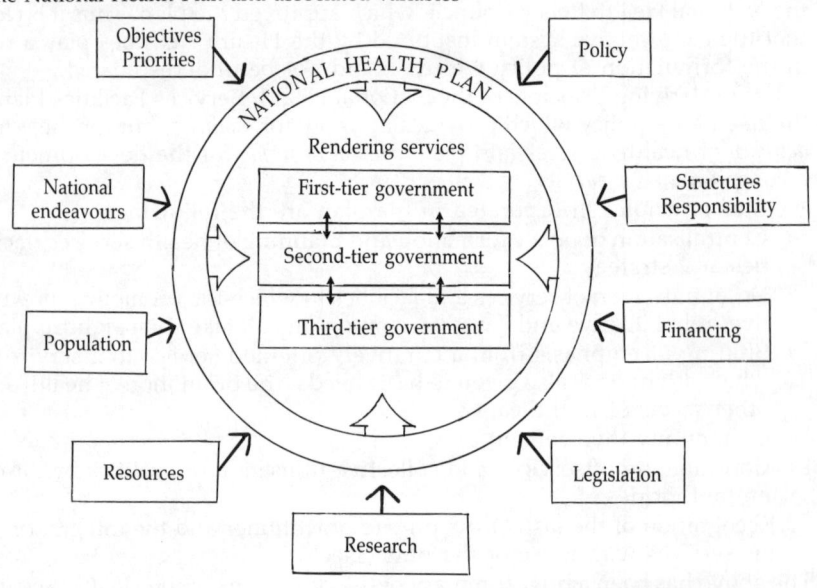

![Diagram: National Health Plan with surrounding variables — Objectives/Priorities, Policy, National endeavours, Structures/Responsibility, Population, Financing, Resources, Legislation, Research — around an inner circle showing Rendering services across First-tier, Second-tier, and Third-tier government.]

The most critical components which have a bearing on the Plan are:
- the national health policy, health objectives and priorities
- the responsibility of the authorities assigned to the rendering of health services
- health financing based on the national health policy, objectives and priorities.

Responsibility for rendering health services

Levels I-III

These are to be managed by:
- the Administrations: House of Assembly
  House of Representatives
  House of Delegates

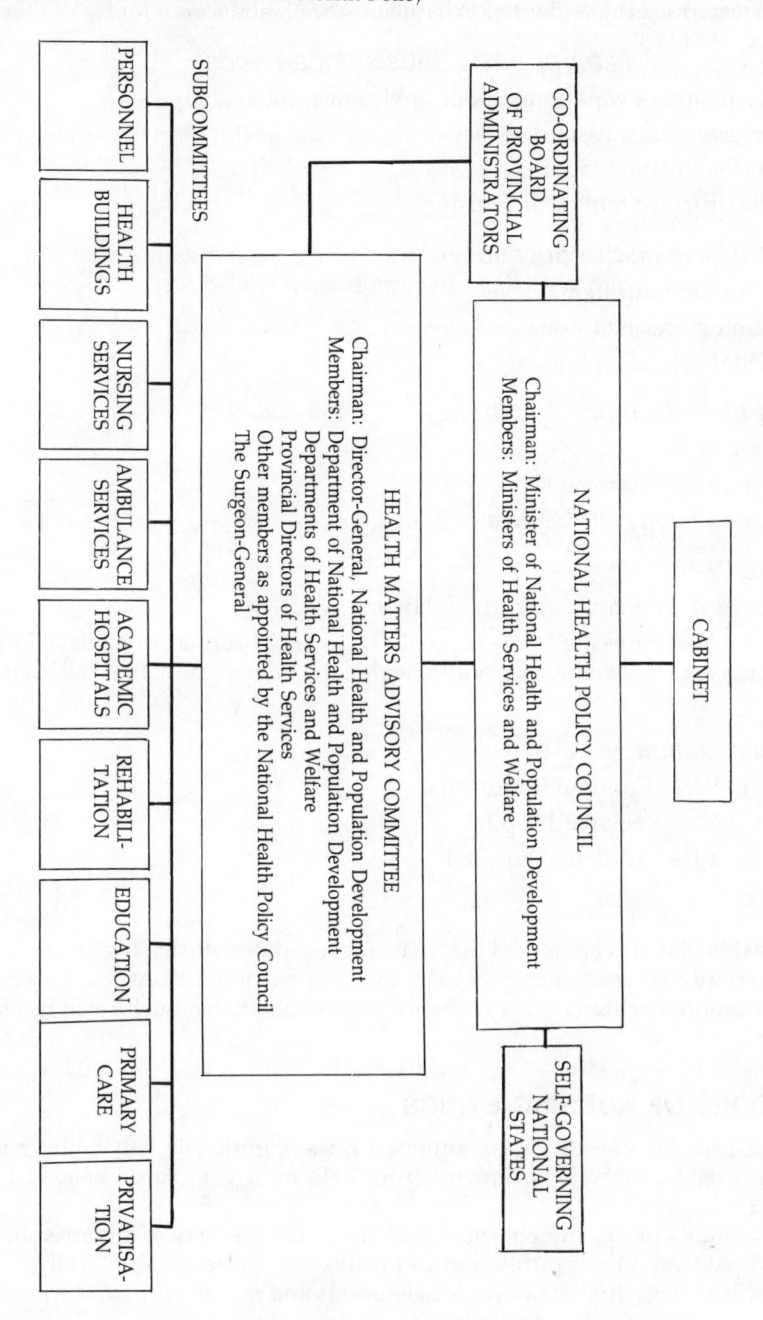

The formulation of the National Health Policy

```
                    ┌─────────────────┐
                    │ CO-ORDINATING   │
                    │     BOARD       │
                    │  OF PROVINCIAL  │
                    │ ADMINISTRATORS  │
                    └────────┬────────┘
                             │
┌──────────────┐    ┌────────┴────────────────────────────────┐
│ PERSONNEL    │    │       NATIONAL HEALTH POLICY COUNCIL    │
├──────────────┤    │                                         │
│ HEALTH       │    │ Chairman: Minister of National Health   │
│ BUILDINGS    │    │          and Population Development     │
├──────────────┤    │ Members: Ministers of Health Services   │
│ NURSING      │    │          and Welfare                    │
│ SERVICES     │    └────────┬────────────────────────────────┘
├──────────────┤             │
│ AMBULANCE    │    ┌────────┴────────────────────────────────┐
│ SERVICES     │    │      HEALTH MATTERS ADVISORY COMMITTEE  │
├──────────────┤    │                                         │
│ ACADEMIC     │────│ Chairman: Director-General, National    │
│ HOSPITALS    │    │   Health and Population Development     │
├──────────────┤    │ Members: Department of National Health  │
│ REHABILI-    │    │   and Population Development            │
│ TATION       │    │   Departments of Health Services and    │
├──────────────┤    │   Welfare                               │
│ EDUCATION    │    │   Provincial Directors of Health        │
├──────────────┤    │   Services                              │
│ PRIMARY      │    │ Other members as appointed by the       │
│ CARE         │    │   National Health Policy Council        │
├──────────────┤    │ The Surgeon-General                     │
│ PRIVATISA-   │    └─────────────────────────────────────────┘
│ TION         │
└──────────────┘
SUBCOMMITTEES
```

CABINET

SELF-GOVERNING NATIONAL STATES

☐ the Department of National Health and Population Development, but for delegated execution by the Provincial Administrations.

Level I – Provision of basic subsistence needs
☐ Safe drinking water and wider environmental health
☐ Sewerage and waste disposal
☐ Food supplementation
☐ Infrastructure and basic housing

Level II – Health education
☐ Minimum educational level
☐ Training and education
☐ Guidance

Level III – Primary health care
☐ Self-care
☐ Community nursing services
☐ Community health centres

Levels IV-VI
These are to be managed in the following way:

Delegated services are to be executed by Provincial Administrations, which also act as agents for other authorities, within the framework of the total health plan.

Hospitalisation
☐ Level IV – Community hospital
☐ Level V – Regional hospital
☐ Level VI – Academic hospital

* * * * *

Under this plan it is envisaged that in future a comprehensive health service will be rendered cost-effectively to all the peoples of South Africa. Preventive, promotive, curative, maintenance and rehabilitative health will be *one service*.

D CODES OF NURSING ETHICS

The *Florence Nightingale Pledge*, although Miss Nightingale had nothing to do with its framing, was drawn up in 1893 by a committee headed by Mrs LE Gretter:

> I solemnly pledge myself before God and in the presence of this assembly;
> To pass my life in purity and to practise my profession faithfully;
> I will abstain from whatever is deleterious and mischievous and will not take or knowingly administer any harmful drug;

I will do all in my power to maintain and elevate the standard of my profession, and will hold in confidence all personal matters committed to my keeping and all family affairs coming to my knowledge in the practice of my calling;
With loyalty will I endeavour to aid the physician in his work, and devote myself to the welfare of those committed to my care.

The *International Code of Nursing Ethics* was adopted by the International Council of Nurses in July 1953 and revised and adopted by the Grand Council Meeting in Frankfurt in June 1965:

Nurses minister to the sick, assume responsibility for creating a physical, social and spiritual environment which will be conducive to recovery, and stress the prevention of illness and promotion of health by teaching and example. They render health service to the individual, the family and the community and coordinate their services with members of other health professions.

Service to mankind is the primary function of nurses and the reason for the existence of the nursing profession. Need for nursing service is universal. Professional nursing service is based on human need and is therefore unrestricted by considerations of nationality, race, creed, colour, politics or social status.

Inherent in the code is the fundamental concept that the nurse believes in the essential freedom of mankind and in the preservation of human life. It is important that all nurses be aware of the Red Cross Principles and of their rights and obligations under the terms of the Geneva Convention of 1949.

The profession recognises that an international code cannot cover in detail all the activities, and relationships of nurses, some of which are conditioned by personal philosophies and beliefs.

1 The fundamental responsibility of the nurse is threefold; to conserve life, to alleviate suffering and to promote health.
2 The nurse shall maintain at all times the highest standards of nursing care and of professional conduct.
3 The nurse must not only be well prepared to practise but shall maintain knowledge and skill at a consistently high level.
4 The religious beliefs of a patient shall be respected.
5 Nurses hold in confidence all personal information entrusted to them.
6 Nurses not only recognise the responsibilities but the limitations of their professional functions; do not recommend or give medical treatment without medical orders except in emergencies, and report such action to a physician as soon as possible.
7 The nurse is under obligation to carry out the physician's orders intelligently and loyally and to refuse to participate in unethical procedures.

8 The nurse sustains confidence in the physician and other members of the health team; incompetence or unethical conduct of associates should be exposed but only to the proper authority. *Fidelity*

9 The nurse is entitled to just remuneration and accepts only such compensation as the contract, actual or implied, provides.

10 Nurses do not permit their names to be used in connection with the advertisement of products or with any other forms of self-advertisement. *Fidelity*

11 The nurse co-operates with and maintains harmonious relationships with members of other professions and with nursing colleagues. *Fidelity*

12 The nurse adheres to standards of personal ethics which reflect credit upon the profession. *Fidelity*

13 In personal conduct nurses should not knowingly disregard the accepted pattern of behaviour of the community in which they live and work. *Veracity / Fidelity*

14 The nurse participates in and shares responsibility with other citizens and health professionals in establishing facilities to meet the health needs of the community and the state, at national and international level. *Ben.*

The *South African Nurses' Pledge of Service* reads as follows:

I solemnly pledge myself to the service of humanity and will endeavour to practise my profession with conscience and with dignity. *Fidelity*

I will maintain by all the means in my power the honour and the noble traditions of my profession. *Fidelity*

The total health of my patients will be my first consideration. *Beneficence / Non maleficence*

I will hold in confidence all personal matters coming to my knowledge.

I will not permit considerations of religion, nationality, race or social standing to intervene between my duty and my patient. *Justice / Autonomy*

I will maintain the utmost respect for human life. *Justice / Autonomy*

I make these promises solemnly, freely and upon my honour.

The *Nurse's Creed* prepared by Ernst van Heerden for the nurses of South Africa reads as follows:

I believe that the honourable profession I am now entering confers on me not only a privilege but also an immense responsibility. I shall endeavour to be worthy of both and to fulfil my duties with dedication and fortitude. In the complex curative organization I hope to aid the physician in my own special and indeed indispensable way.

Compassion for my patients will be the lodestar of my life, for without a sense of pity and generosity my work will become merely an impersonal mechanical trade.

That is why I propose to make my own contribution – small though it might be – towards the humanizing of our art, towards the spiritual and physical needs of those placed in my care.

I am intensely aware of the vulnerability of man and the frail structure which the human body is. That I am able to apply myself to the amelioration of suffering, consolation in sorrow and assurance in despair; these are the sources of my gratitude and joy.

I see myself as the sounding-board for my patients in their discomfort, pain and fear and I shall at all times consider them as individuals with their own special qualities and needs. Each one of them is to me an embodiment of the wonder of life which it is my duty in all humility to sustain.

I shall devote myself to the maintenance of the highest standards in my profession, to respecting the norms and values set by my teachers.

At all times I wish to bear in mind the example of the noble women who preceded me and hope that I too may be for many 'the lady with the lamp', a beacon in a world of darkness and suffering.

Ultimately I see my work as an expression of love, a love that transcends differences of race, creed, religion and social standing. So may my daily striving embody a universal truth – that of faith, hope and charity, and the greatest of these is charity.

The UKCC has also drawn up a code and the Rcn has drawn up a discussion document on professional and personal responsibility. The address of the United Kingdom Central Council for Nursing, Midwifery and Health Visiting (PC division) is 23 Portland Place, London W1N 3AF, and the address of the Rcn is The Royal College of Nursing of the United Kingdom, Henrietta Place, London W1M 0AB.

The documents make interesting reading and are recommended to serious students of nursing. They emphasise the nurse's duty to patients, the existence of different customs and religious beliefs among different groups, the importance of avoiding harm to patients and the need for nurses to maintain professional competence and accept and acknowledge any limitations of competence. Nurses work as members of a team, respect confidential information and assist others to gain competence. It will be seen that codes of professional conduct drawn up by various bodies have a high degree of similarity.

E CRITERIA FOR BRAIN DEATH

Minimum criteria for a diagnosis of brain death[1]

The diagnosis of brain death can only be made if the answer to *all* the questions is *no*.

1 Cooper & Lanza 1984: 38.

1 Respiration*
   (a) Is there spontaneous ventilation within 5 minutes of disconnecting the ventilator (with P_aCO_2 normal before the ventilator was disconnected)?
   or
   (b) Is there any spontaneous ventilation within 10 minutes of disconnecting the ventilator?

2 Brain stem reflexes
   (a) Do the pupils react to light?
       Do the pupils react to painful stimulation?
   (b) Are doll's eye movements present?
   (c) Does nystagmus occur when each ear is in turn irrigated with ice-cold water for 1 minute?
   (d) Is there any movement in the head and neck, either spontaneously or in response to stimulation?
   (e) Is there a gag or a reflex response following bronchial stimulation by a suction catheter passed down the trachea?

3 Body temperature
   Is the rectal temperature below 35°C?

4 Drugs
   Have any drugs which may affect ventilation or the level of consciousness been administered during the past 12 hours?

5 Cerebral state
   Have you any doubt that this patient's cerebral state is due to an irreversible cause?

DATE: .... DOCTOR ....

* Details of testing for spontaneous respiration are given on the reverse of this form.

F ETHICAL GUIDELINES

Declaration of Geneva[2]

(Adopted by WMA at its General Assembly 1948, revised 1968.)

At the time of being admitted as a member of the Medical Profession: I solemnly pledge myself to consecrate my life to the service of humanity; I will give to my teachers the respect and gratitude which is their due; I will practise my profession with conscience and dignity; The health of my patient will be my first consideration; I will respect the secrets which are confided in me, even after the patient has died; I will maintain by

2 Scorer & Wing 1979: 193.

all the means in my power, the honour and the noble traditions of the medical profession; My colleagues will be my brothers; I will not permit considerations of religion, nationality, race, party politics or social standing to intervene between my duty and my patient; I will maintain the utmost respect for human life from the time of conception; even under threat, I will not use my medical knowledge contrary to the laws of humanity. I make these promises solemnly, freely and upon my honour.

Declaration of Helsinki

(Recommendations guiding doctors in clinical research. Adopted by the World Medical Assembly, Helsinki, Finland, 1964.)

Introduction

It is the mission of the doctor to safeguard the health of the people. His knowledge and conscience are dedicated to the fulfilment of this mission.

The Declaration of Geneva of The World Medical Association binds the doctor with the words: 'The health of my patient will be my first consideration' and the International Code of Medical Ethics which declares that 'Any act or advice which could weaken physical or mental resistance of a human being may be used only in his interest.'

Because it is essential that the results of laboratory experiments be applied to human beings to further scientific knowledge and to help suffering humanity, The World Medical Association has prepared the following recommendations as a guide to each doctor in clinical research. It must be stressed that the standards as drafted are only a guide to physicians all over the world. Doctors are not relieved from criminal, civil and ethical responsibilities under the laws of their own countries.

In the field of clinical research a fundamental distinction must be recognized between clinical research in which the aim is essentially therapeutic for a patient, and clinical research, the essential object of which is purely scientific and without therapeutic value to the person subjected to the research.

1 Basic principles

1. Clinical research must conform to the moral and scientific principles that justify medical research and should be based on laboratory and animal experiments or other scientifically established facts.
2. Clinical research should be conducted only by scientifically qualified persons and under the supervision of a qualified medical man.
3. Clinical research cannot legitimately be carried out unless the importance of the objective is in proportion to the inherent risk to the subject.
4. Every clinical research project should be preceded by careful assessment of inherent risks in comparison to foreseeable benefits to the subject or to others.

5 Special caution should be exercised by the doctor in performing clinical research in which the personality of the subject is liable to be altered by drugs or experimental procedure.

II Clinical research combined with professional care

1 In the treatment of the sick person, the doctor must be free to use a new therapeutic measure, if in his judgement it offers hope of saving life, re-establishing health, or alleviating suffering.

   If at all possible, consistent with patient psychology, the doctor should obtain the patient's freely given consent after the patient has been given a full explanation. In case of legal incapacity, consent should also be procured from the legal guardian; in case of physical incapacity the permission of the legal guardian replaces that of the patient.

2 The doctor can combine clinical research with professional care, the objective being the acquisition of new medical knowledge, only to the extent that clinical research is justified by its therapeutic value for the patient.

III Non-therapeutic clinical research

1 In the purely scientific application of clinical research carried out on a human being, it is the duty of the doctor to remain the protector of the life and health of that person on whom clinical research is being carried out.

2 The nature, the purpose and the risk of clinical research must be explained to the subject by the doctor.

3a Clinical research on a human being cannot be undertaken without his free consent after he has been informed; if he is legally incompetent, the consent of the legal guardian should be procured.

3b The subject of clinical research should be in such a mental, physical and legal state as to be able to exercise fully his power of choice.

3c Consent should, as a rule, be obtained in writing. However, the responsibility for clinical research always remains with the research worker; it never falls on the subject even after consent is obtained.

4a The investigator must respect the right of each individual to safeguard his personal integrity, especially if the subject is in a dependent relationship to the investigator.

4b At any time during the course of clinical research the subject or his guardian should be free to withdraw permission for research to be continued.

The investigator or the investigating team should discontinue the research if in his or their judgement, it may, if continued, be harmful to the individual.

Bibliography

ACTS

Nursing Act, 1978 (Act 50 of 1978), as amended by Act 71 of 1981.

ARTICLES, BROCHURES AND PAPERS

Beaton, GR & Bourne, DE. 1980. Trends in the distribution of Medical Manpower in South Africa. *SA Medical Journal*, 17 May.

Cooper, DKC, DeVilliers, JC, Smith, LS, Crombie, Y, Boyd, ST, Jacobson, JE & Barnard, CN. 1982. Medical, legal and administrative aspects of cadaveric donation in the RSA. *SA Medical Journal*, 62.

Department of Health. 1986. *A new dispensation: health services in South Africa*, Pretoria: Government Printer.

Dixon, E. 1982. The first international congress on nursing law and ethics. *Guy's Hospital Gazette*, 96(2325).

Hirschfeld, MJ. 1985. Ethics and care for the Elderly. *International journal of nursing studies*, 22(4).

Levine, M. 1978. Paper given at the Conference for Nurse Educators, New York. 3-6 December.

Mellish, JM. 1984. Primary health care – the role of the nurse. *Curationis*, March.

Poletti, RA. 1985. Ethics of death and dying. *International journal of nursing studies*, 22(4).

Rip, MR, Roux, AJ & Roberts, MM. 1986. Birth and fertility rate, variations in metropolitan Cape Town. *The SA journal of epidemiology and infection*.

Searle, C. 1982. The dependent, interdependent and independent functions of the nurse practitioner – A legal and ethical aspect. *Curationis*, December.

Smith, SJ & Davis, AJ. 1985. A programme for nursing ethics. *International journal of nursing studies*, 22(4).

SA Nursing Association. 1985. *A guide for members*. SANA.

Woodruff, AM. 1985. Becoming a nurse: the ethical perspective. *International journal of nursing studies*, 22(4).

BOOKS

Baly, ME. 1984. *Professional Responsibility*. 2nd ed. London: Wiley.

Benatar, SR. (Ed). 1986. *Ethical and moral issues in contemporary medical practice*. Proceedings of a University of Cape Town Faculty of Medicine Symposium, 1985. Cape Town: UCT publication.

Carr-Saunders, AM & Wilson, PA. 1933. *The Professions*. London: Frank Cass and Co Ltd.
Cooper, DKC & Lanza, RP. (Eds). 1984. *Heart transplantation*. Lancaster: MTP Press Ltd.
Donahue, MP. 1985. *Nursing, the finest art*. St Louis: CV Mosby Co.
Guide to the Health Act, No 63 of 1977. Pretoria: Government Printer, 1978.
Hockey, Lisbeth. (Ed). 1981. *Recent advances in nursing. Current Issues in nursing*. Edinburgh: Churchill Livingstone.
King, I. 1971. *Toward a theory for nursing*. New York: Wiley.
Kozier, B & Erb, G. 1982. *Techniques in clinical nursing*. California: Addison-Wesley Publishing Co.
Lysaught, J. 1970. *An Abstract for Action*. New York: McGraw-Hill.
Mellish, JM. 1984. *A basic history of nursing*. Durban: Butterworths.
Myles, M. 1981. *Textbook for midwives*. 9th ed. Edinburgh: Churchill Livingstone.
Rothwell, NV. 1977. *Human Genetics*. Englewood Cliffs, NJ: Prentice-Hall.
Schulberg, L. 1966. Historic India. *Great Ages of Man*. The Netherlands: Time-Life International.
Scorer, G & Wing, A. (Eds). 1979. *Decision making in medicine: the practice of its ethics*. London: Edward Arnold.
Searle, C. 1965. *History of the Development of nursing in South Africa*. Pretoria: SANA.
Searle, C & Brink, H. 1982. *Aspects of Community Health*. 5th ed. Cape Town: King Edward VII Trust.
Strauss, SA. 1981. *Legal handbook for nurses and health personnel*. Cape Town: King Edward VII Trust.
Walker, EA. 1968. *A History of Southern Africa*. London: Longmans, Green & Co Ltd.
Woodham-Smith, C. 1951. *Florence Nightingale*. New York: McGraw-Hill.

REGULATIONS/RULES SA NURSING COUNCIL

Government Notice R 387. 15 Feb 1985. Rules setting out the acts and omissions in respect of which the Council may take disciplinary steps. Pretoria: Government Printer.
Government Notice R 2598. 14 Nov 1984. As amended by R1469, 10 July 1987. Regulations relating to the scope of practice of persons who are registered or enrolled under the Act. Pretoria: Government Printer.

REPORTS

Joint Report WHO and UNICEF to Alma-Ata Conference, September 1978.
Wessels, J. 1983. *A progress report of primary health care in the Eastern Cape and Border, 1979-1982*.

Index

A

Abortion 125-126
Acts
 Abortion and Sterilisation 126
 Health 58, 59, 60
 Human tissue 121
 Medical 45, 89, 90, 166
 Mental Health 52
 Nursing 35, 63, 76, 77, 90, 92, 97
 Public Health 58, 59
 South Africa 31
Accoucheur/male midwife 46
Accountability 74, 93, 140-147
Afrikaanse Christelike
 Vrouevereniging 30, 57
Afrikaner nation 29, 51
Ageing population 118
Alexander, BG 28, 29
Alma-Ata Conference 60
American system 163-164
Analytic ethics 106
Anglican sisters 16, 17, 27
Anglo-Boer War 28, 30
Artificial insemination 127-128
Attitude of mind 136-137
Attitude to health care 19-20
Auxiliary midwives 47
Auxiliary nurses 34-35
Autonomy 108

B

Beneficience 109
Black nurses 15, 28, 33-35
Black nations 27, 32-37
Brain death, criteria for 187-188
British 26-29
Brownlee, J 32, 33
Buddhism 14, 115

C

Cadaver donation 120-121
Cecilia Makiwane 34
Chamberlens 41
Christianity 15-16, 53-54, 72, 110, 114-115, 157, 164
Chronic illness and the nurse 174
Codes of ethics 140, 184-187
 (Appendix D)
Coding system for resuscitation 123
Colleagues 132-133
Colleges of nursing 167
Coloured group 36, 37-38
Community nursing 19, 52-60, 167, 168
Compassion 137
Composition of nursing profession 82-84
Comprehensive nursing 2, 167-168
Computers 118
Conflict of duty 138-139
Conflict in work situation 117-130
Continental system 164-165
Cost factors 117-118, 119
Crises 174-175
Criteria for brain death 187-188
 (Appendix E)
Criteria for a profession 70-82

D

De Beer 31, 165
Declarations
 Geneva 107, 110, 129, 188
  (Appendix F)
 Helsinki 107, 128, 129, 189-191
  (Appendix F)
 Human rights 175
 Sydney 120
Degrees in nursing 169-170
Dependent function 92-93

Descriptive ethics 104
Discipline 148-155
Disciplinary control 89, 90, 91, 94, 95, 96, 140
Dix 49
Dunant 17
Dutch East India Co 26, 44, 50
Dutch settlement 26
Duty 131-139
  to clients/patients 131-132
  to colleagues 132-133
  to employer 135-136
  to fellow men 131-132
  to herself 133-135
  to profession 133
  conflict of 138-139

E

Education, nursing 4, 5, 23, 24, 65, 160-170
Enrolled nurses 25, 40, 170
Environmental factors 19, 22
Ethics 12, 104-130, 184-187
Ethical problems 110-130
Ethos 1, 12
Euthanasia 115, 121-124
Evolving role of nurse 1, 2, 24-25, 115-116
Exploration and colonisation 18

F

Family planning 62, 126-127
Fitzgerald, Dr 33, 34
Fliedner 161
Florence Nightingale 17, 21, 39, 54, 73, 77, 158, 161, 162
Functions of nurse
  dependent 12, 13
  independent 12-13
  interdependent 12-13
First hospital 27

G

Genetics 125
General nursing 39-40

Geneva declaration 107, 110, 129, 188 (Appendix F)
Greeks 15, 41, 53

H

Health 171-176
Health Act 58, 59, 60
Health education 62-63
Health Matters Advisory Committee 178-179
Hebrews 14-15, 41, 53
Heidelberg University 22, 160
Hinduism 14
Hippocrates 22, 41
Hippocratic Oath 15, 107, 108, 177 (Appendix A)
History 1, 12-38
Hobhouse, E 28
Hospitals
  Albany 27, 51
  Baragwanath 64, 169
  Barberton 27, 165
  Bond van Afrikaanse Moeders 30
  Carnarvon 27, 165
  Frontier 165
  Groote Schuur 37, 166
  Johannesburg 169
  Kimberley 165, 166
  Lovedale 34, 37
  McCord Zulu 34
  Somerset 26, 50, 165
  Tygerberg 37

I

Independent functions of nurse 91-92
Interdependent functions of nurse 91, 92
Indian nurses 36
In-service education 68, 69, 81
Inspection 151
International Code of Ethics 185-186
International Council of Nurses 88, 185
In vitro fertilisation 127-128

J

Jan van Riebeeck 26, 144
Judaism 14, 107, 114

K

Kaiserwerth 161

L

Lamp, symbolism of 10-11
Le Gras 49, 54
Living will 122
Loopuyt 31
Lotz, E 31

M

Machines 2, 117
Makiwane, C 34
Male midwife 46
Mary Agatha, sister 165
May, Dr Franz 22, 160
Medical crises and the nurse 174-175
Medical councils
  Colonial 34, 37, 46, 165
  South African 63, 86, 90, 97
  Supreme Medical Committee 26, 45
Medical ethics 107-108
Military nursing 16, 17, 27
Missions 32-34, 58-59
Motherhouse system 164

N

Natalse Christelike Vrouevereniging 30, 57
National Health Policy Council 177-178 (Appendix B)
National Health Services Plan 65, 181, 182-184
Nightingale, F 17, 21, 39, 54, 73, 77, 158, 161, 162
Nightingale System/School 22, 34, 161, 162-163, 165
Normative ethics 105-106

Nursing
  Act 35, 63, 76, 77, 90, 92, 97
  administration 156-160
  as a profession 78-88
  community 19, 52-60
  courses
    post-basic/post-registration
      Administration 168
      Community 168, 169
      Education 168, 169, 170
      Geriatric 68, 169
      Intensive 68
      In-service 68, 69, 81
      Oncology 168
      Operating Theatre 68, 168
      Ophthalmic 68, 168
      Orthopaedic 68, 168
      Paediatric 68, 168
      Spinal injury 168
      Renal 168
  definition 9-10
  education 4, 5, 23, 24, 65, 160-170
  ethics 106-107 184-187
  general 39-40
  occupational health 55, 59, 65
  psychiatric 49-52
  registration 27, 51
  research 23, 118-119, 128-130
  what it is 1-11

O

Occupational health 55, 59, 65
Oranje Vrouevereniging 30, 57
Organ transplantation 119-121

P

Parsons, E 33
Philosophical approach 109
Pinel, P 46
Pledge of service 10, 186
Power 115-117
Preventive and promotive health care 23, 43, 62
Priest physicians 13
Primary health care 60-66, 116
Privatisation 66

Problems, ethical 110-130
Products of conception 127
Profession 70-88
Professional association 84-88
Professional ethics 106-108
Professional practice 89-98, 101-103
Psychiatric nursing 49-52

Q

Quality of life 111-113

R

Red Cross 17
Religion 12-16, 29-30, 70, 72, 124
Religious orders 16, 88
Research 23, 118-119, 128-130
Rights and responsibilities 111, 113, 175-176
Rome, Romans, Roman matrons 16, 41, 53

S

Sanctity of life 110-111
School nurse 59, 65
Scientific and technological developments 7, 21-24, 67, 118, 146, 157
Searle, C 9, 31, 70, 89, 91, 96, 169
Sickness and society 172-174
Social change 18-21, 108
Space medicine 1, 23
Specialisation 66-69
South African
 Act 31
 Medical Council 63, 86, 90, 97, 166, 167
 Nursing Association 36, 85, 86, 93, 97-101
 Nursing Council 9, 36, 40, 51, 68, 75, 76, 77, 80, 83, 84, 86, 90, 93-96, 140, 166, 168, 170
 Trained Nurses' Association 76, 85, 97
Vrouefederasie 30, 57

Status of women 20-21
Stockdale, Sister Henrietta 16, 27, 45, 46, 165, 166
Students 141, 144-145
Subprofessional groups 170
Supervision 149, 150-151
Supreme Medical Committee 26, 45
Surrogate mothers 127-128

T

Team approach 2, 68, 69, 133
Technology 7, 21-24, 67, 118, 146, 157
Theories of nursing 11
Therapeutic use of self 4, 5, 10
Traditional birth attendants 47
Transplants, organ 119-121
Triage 123
Truth telling/veracity 109, 113-115

U

University education for nurses 35, 164
University link with nursing colleges 167

V

Van Riebeeck 26, 44
Vincent de Paul 49, 54, 160
Voluntary organisations 57-58

W

Wars 16-18
Watkins, MH 45, 46
Wehr, Dr 44-45
World Health Organisation 60, 171
World Medical Association 120, 128
Well-being 137-138

196